Fabricated or Induced Illness in a Child by a Carer

A Reader

Christopher Bools
Consultant Child and Adolescent Psychiatrist

Radcliffe Publishing
Oxford ● New York

Radcliffe Publishing Ltd
18 Marcham Road
Abingdon
Oxon OX14 1AA
United Kingdom

www.radcliffe-oxford.com
Electronic catalogue and worldwide online ordering facility.

British Library Cataloguing in Publication Data

A catalogue record for this book is available from the British Library.

ISBN-13: 978 1 84619 134 3

Typeset by Advance Typesetting Ltd, Oxford
Printed and bound by Biddles Ltd, King's Lynn, Norfolk

Contents

Introduction to the training materials

Statement of purpose

We have moved beyond recognition and description of the rare forms of child abuse now referred to as *Fabricated Illness* or *Induced Illness* (FII). The purpose of these training materials, of which this *Reader* is one part, is to contribute to the ongoing development of multi-disciplinary, multi-agency work, which will safeguard and promote the welfare of the children who have had illness fabricated or induced. Critically this will include work with parents and carers. The training materials support the Government Guidance on FII first issued in 2002 and updated in 2007.

Development of the training materials

A group of professionals, from a variety of professional backgrounds, gathered together to produce training materials under the direction of the DfES through 2004 to 2006.

The training materials consist of:

- Training Exercises
- PowerPoint presentations
- Film (scenarios on a DVD)
- Reader
- Trainer's Introduction and Guide.

About the Reader

Attention has been given to presenting information under headings covering similar areas of interest in both this *Reader* and in the *Training Exercises*. After watching the *Training Film*, and participating in selected exercises at a training session, the professional may wish to study topics in more depth. The author's intention is to assist the busy professional by providing easy access to summarized accounts of original sources of information, including experiences of professionals and victims of FII, as an additional evidence base for practice. Alternatively the *Reader* may be studied before attending a training session and also referred to anytime, as the need arises.

The steering group

- Christopher Bools, Consultant in Child and Adolescent Psychiatry, Avon and Wiltshire Partnership NHS Trust.
- Mary Eminson, Consultant in Child and Adolescent Psychiatry, Bolton Hospitals NHS Trust.
- John Fox, former Detective Inspector, Hampshire Police Authority.
- Jenny Gray, Professional Advisor, DfES London.
- Jan Horwath, Professor of Social Policy, University of Sheffield.
- Margaret Lynch, Emeritus Professor of Community Paediatrics, King's College London.
- Richard Wilson, Emeritus Consultant in Paediatrics, Kingston Hospital NHS Trust.

Thanks for advice to Arnon Bentovim, Consultant in Child and Family Psychiatry, London Child and Family Consultation Centre, and David Jones, Consultant in Child and Family Psychiatry, Honorary Senior Lecturer, University of Oxford, Park Hospital for Children, Oxford.

Chapter 1

Overview

Section headings
What is Fabricated or Induced Illness (FII)?
Statement on definition
Statement re: nomenclature
KEY WORDS/PHRASES
Fabricated or Induced Illness (FII)
Munchausen Syndrome by Proxy (MSbP/MSP)

What is Fabricated or Induced Illness (FII)?
Statement on definition

Essentially Fabricated or Induced Illness (FII) is a descriptive term and therefore substantially defines itself. A wide range of situations is potentially covered by the term and a representative variety is presented in Chapter 2. The history, and controversy, about the use of the term MSbP was discussed in the *Report of the RCPCH Working Party* published in 2002, which recommended that paediatricians should talk about *Fabricated or Induced Illness*. In the Government Guidance *Safeguarding Children in Whom Illness is Fabricated or Induced* (Department of Health *et al.*, 2002, section 1.4), the point is made that differences of opinion about terminology, and the use of various terms, may result in the loss of focus on the welfare of the child. In referring to 'fabrication or induction of illness in a child' the primary focus of professional activity is directed upon the welfare (health and development) and safety of the child.

In addition, it is intended that the use of the descriptive term FII discourages a tendency for the situation to be viewed as a discrete medical syndrome, which it is not. Use of the term FII sidesteps the process of considering complicated 'diagnostic criteria' which require consideration of both what happens to the child (*see* Chapters 2 and 5) in combination with the psychiatric status of the fabricator (*see* Chapter 4). However, consideration of both of these elements of FII will be important in deciding upon the course of management (discussed in Chapters 6 to 9). Whilst a range of behaviours displayed by a suspected fabricator may be useful in raising concerns, only the certainty of fabrication, or induction, of illness itself is the critical evidence for applying the term FII to a situation. This decision will usually be made by a paediatrician functioning as part of a multi-disciplinary team.

Whilst it is usually fairly clear, or at least open to clarifying medical investigation, when illness is being induced in a child, difficulties sometimes arise when professionals are unclear if the parent is fabricating, exaggerating, or merely highly anxious about their child. Thus it is helpful to consider such uncertainties within an approach which considers the illness state of the child, the psychological state of the parent in relation to the child, and the behaviour of the parent with the child within the healthcare system. FII is looked at this way in Chapter 3. This approach should be taken within the context of the three domains of the Assessment Framework set out in paragraph 5.37 of *Working Together to Safeguard Children* (HM Government, 2006) and revisited in Chapter 3 of *Safeguarding Children in Whom Illness is Fabricated or Induced* (HM Government, 2007). To recap, the three domains are: the child's developmental needs, parenting capacity, and family and environmental factors.

Statement re: nomenclature

Both the Government Guidance and the Royal College of Paediatrics and Child Health Report recommend using the term *'Fabrication or Induction of Illness in a Child'* (FII). Other terms have been used to refer to the situation when illness has been fabricated or induced and their appropriateness has been debated. Most commonly the term *MSP* (or MSbP) has been used. This may result in lack of clarity (even confusion), especially if this term is misapplied to the perpetrator as a psychiatric diagnosis (*see* section 1 of the Government Guidance). In addition, the term *MSP* was derived from the term *Munchausen Syndrome*, which has been used to refer to a disorder of adults who chronically fabricate illnesses in themselves and often travel from one hospital to another to present themselves to new medical teams, sometimes in the context of a wandering lifestyle and maybe even homelessness. It has been argued that the term *Munchausen Syndrome* itself is anachronistic, and potentially misleading, and in practice it has probably been largely replaced by the term *Factitious Disorder*. Following the identification of the fabrication or induction of illness in a child, the question of any psychiatric diagnosis applicable to the perpetrator is usually a secondary, although important consideration. Nevertheless, despite the recommended use of this terminology, in order to access information about FII it has been necessary to examine literature which mostly has the term MSP in the title – as the term has been in widespread use over the period from 1976 before the current recommendation was made.

Other terms have been used by workers to refer to situations which are on the spectrum of situations discussed in Chapter 3. Some of these may include examples also appropriately labelled as FII; however, each example would need to be considered on its own merits. Examples of terms found in medical literature are 'doctor shopping with the child as proxy patient' (Woollcott *et al.*, 1982), 'peregrinating pediatric patient' (Fialkov, 1984), 'extreme illness exaggeration in pediatric patients' (Masterson, Dunworth and Williams, 1988) 'the persistent parent' (Waring, 1992), and 'outlandish factitious illness' (Taylor, 1992).

References

Department of Health, Home Office, Department for Education and Skills, Welsh Assembly Government. *Safeguarding Children in Whom Illness is Fabricated or Induced.* London: Department of Health Publications; 2002.

Fialkov MJ. Peregrination in the problem pediatric patient: the pediatric Munchausen syndrome? *Clinical Pediatrics.* 1984; 23(10): 571–5.

HM Government. *Working Together to Safeguard Children: a guide for interagency working to safeguard and promote the welfare of children.* London: The Stationery Office; 2006.

HM Government. *Safeguarding Children in Whom Illness is Fabricated or Induced.* London: Department for Education and Skills; 2007. www.everychildmatters. gov.uk/safeguarding

Masterson J, Dunworth R, Williams N. Extreme illness exaggeration in pediatric patients: a variant of Munchausen's by proxy? *American Journal of Orthopsychiatry.* 1988; 58(2): 188–95.

Royal College of Paediatrics and Child Health. *Fabricated or Induced Illness by Carers.* London: Royal College of Paediatrics and Child Health; February 2002. www.rcpch.ac.uk

Taylor DC. Outlandish Factitious Illness. In: David TJ, editor. *Recent Advances in Paediatrics.* Edinburgh: Churchill Livingstone; 1992. 10: 63–76.

Waring WW. The persistent parent. *American Journal of Diseases in Childhood.* 1992; 146: 753–6.

Woollcott P, Aceto T, Rutt C, Bloom M, Glick R. Doctor shopping with the child as proxy patient: a variant of child abuse. *Journal of Pediatrics*. 1982; **101**(2): 297–301.

Further reading

Bentovim A. A 20-year overview. In: Adshead G, Brooke D, editors. *Munchausen's Syndrome by Proxy. Current issues in assessment, treatment and research*. London: Imperial College Press; 2001.

Department of Health, Department for Education and Employment and the Home Office. *Framework for the Assessment of Children in Need and their Families*. London: The Stationery Office; 2000.

Eminson M. Munchausen syndrome by proxy – an introduction. In: Eminson M, Postlethwaite RJ, editors. *Munchausen Syndrome by Proxy Abuse: a practical approach*. Oxford: Butterworth Heinemann; 2000. Out of print but pdf available on *Incredibly Caring*. Oxford: Radcliffe Publishing; 2007.

Chapter 2

Nature of the phenomena

Section headings
Presentations of FII
Thirteen examples to illustrate presentations of FII
Verbal fabrications
Falsification of specimens
Illness induction
A possible fabricated psychiatric disorder
Fabrication in the setting of genuine physical illness
Presentations in obstetric settings
Symptom coaching
Examples of participation by the child
KEY WORDS/PHRASES
Verbal fabrication
Fabrication with falsification of specimens or records
Illness induction
Failure to thrive
Factitious Disorder in pregnancy (Obstetric Factitious Disorder)
Symptom coaching

Presentations of FII

There are three main ways in which a carer may fabricate, or induce, illness in a child (HM Government, 2007). These are:

1 Fabrication of signs and symptoms. This may include fabrication of past medical history.
2 Fabrication of signs and symptoms, and falsification of hospital charts and records, and specimens of bodily fluids. This may include falsification of letters and documents.
3 Induction of illness by a variety of means.

It is also useful to note three situations, which are perhaps less obvious, in which FII may occur:

A   Fabrication of psychiatric disorder (a form of verbal fabrication).
B   Fabrication in the presence of genuine physical illness (may be verbal fabrication, falsification, or induction).
C   A Factitious Disorder in the mother related to an aspect of the pregnancy (usually verbal, although rarely may

be illness induction, such as antepartum bleeding, potentially leading to harm to the foetus).

Verbal fabrication (of the history only) is probably the most common and, perhaps, the most difficult situation in which to decide if it is fabrication. It may be less difficult, having gathered the evidence, to decide if the situations of falsification and illness induced are present.

Thirteen examples to illustrate presentations of FII

Table 2.1   Presentations of FII

Verbal	Falsification (falsified specimens or records)	Induction of illness (production of signs)
Apnoea with fit [Croft and Jervis, 1989]	Bleeding [Lee, 1979]	Poisoning [Rogers et al., 1976]
Allergies [Warner and Hathaway, 1984]	Sputum (in CF) [Orenstein and Wasserman, 1986]	Diarrhoea laxatives [Epstein et al., 1987]
Asthma [Roth, 1990]	Diabetes [Nading and Duval-Arnould, 1984]	Smothering [Rosen et al., 1986]
Developmental disorder [Stevenson and Alexander, 1990]	Vomiting [McGuire and Feldman, 1989]	Skin rash [Jones, 1983]
		Failure to thrive by withholding food [Gray and Bentovim, 1996]

Verbal fabrications

Epileptic fits (Croft and Jervis, 1989)

From the age of four years a boy repeatedly feigned epileptic fits. He later admitted that his mother had taught him that he was epileptic and had trained him to behave like that. The boy had been treated with medication for epilepsy for three months. By the age of five years the GP reported that there had been

130 visits to his surgery. In addition, there had been 35 visits to the Accident and Emergency department at the hospital.

Allergies (Warner and Hathaway, 1984)

Seventeen children, from 11 families, were subjected to bizarre diets and lifestyles. The mothers believed that their children had severe allergies to foods and in one case house dust mites: they insisted on many medical consultations. The 17 children had attended a specialist allergy clinic. In all, approximately 1,600 children had attended the clinic at the time and, of these, 301 children had received detailed dietetic assessment for presumed food allergy or intolerance.

The children presented with a variety of symptoms, which the mothers falsely believed were due to food allergy. The majority were behavioural problems, nausea and abdominal pains, asthma, migraine, bed-wetting, epilepsy, rhinitis and diarrhoea. The authors noted that all but two of the children had seen a number of specialists and often the mothers had had vehement disagreements with the consultants. It was observed that 10 of the mothers insisted upon very close involvement with every aspect of their child's life whilst on the ward, which the authors described as exhibiting 'a limpet like attachment to their children'.

With regard to outcomes for the children, despite evidence to the contrary, the beliefs often continued and the children remained on diets and failed allergy clinic follow-up. Seven children had excessive and inappropriate school absences. The outcome for only three of the children was considered to be totally satisfactory, with permanent relaxation of the dietary restrictions and continued follow-up at the clinic.

Asthma (Roth, 1990)

A 10-year-old girl developed a slight cough shortly after her mother was diagnosed with breast cancer. The mother claimed that this was an attack of asthma requiring urgent medical treatment. When the mother was informed that her daughter's cough was not caused by asthma, she would not accept this. She then went from doctor to doctor repeating the asthma claim and demanding medication. One physician prescribed bronchodilators to be used in minimal doses only when needed. However, the mother administered the medication on a regular basis at maximal dose.

Developmental disability (Stevenson and Alexander, 1990)

An 11-month-old girl was presented by the mother as suffering from cerebral palsy, gastrostomy dependence and feeding problems. There was a history of *failure to thrive* at 15 weeks. On examination and following extensive testing in a team assessment, the conclusion was of a child with normal development although with a well-healed gastrostomy scar evident; a picture incongruent with the history presented by the mother. During hospitalization, medical work-up demonstrated no abnormalities with no evidence of seizures and no difficulties with feeding. On four occasions when the mother was unobserved with the child she reported vomiting. The mother was eventually recognized by staff who recalled that she had presented the subject's older sibling with a history of what they refer to as 'near-miss SIDS' (sudden infant death syndrome), vomiting and gastro-oesophageal reflux. This had led to surgery (Nissen fundoplication) despite minimal objective findings and normal growth. Later the mother had continued to report vomiting and worried that the child was suffering from cerebral palsy. It emerged that the mother had a history of hospital admissions with no cause having been found for her own symptoms.

Falsification of specimens

Bleeding (Lee, 1979)

Twin infants had repeated admissions to hospital because the mother reported they were coughing up blood. There were six admissions in the first four months of life. By identifying blood groups, the blood found on the children was eventually proven to originate from the mother.

Simulation of cystic fibrosis (Orenstein and Wasserman, 1986)

A mother, who claimed to be a nurse, presented her child of five years to a cystic fibrosis (CF) clinic with a history consistent with that disorder; aspects of the history were later found to have been falsified. On examination of the child in hospital, the child was poorly nourished and there were signs of disease in one lung (atelactasis and perhaps bronchiectasis but not CF). Although the mother reported that the child had raised sodium chloride in a sweat test carried out at age five months she would not permit this test to be carried out. Over a year later the child was re-admitted to hospital for treatments of chest infections and cough, which were always relieved by antibiotics.

Eventually special tests for CF were carried out; it was shown that the mother altered sweat tests and claimed that it was not possible to collect stools for fat analyses. She also took sputum from other children who genuinely suffered from the disorder and presented the specimens as if they had come from her own child. A direct examination of the lungs by bronchoscopy indicated that disease was limited to the right lower lobe only (the problem was narrowing of the opening to 30% of normal and there was no evidence of CF). The mother was informed that the bronchoscopy had shown a much better picture than could have been hoped for with most children with CF.

At this point the mother herself experienced various symptoms and took to her child's hospital bed. Later, when she was informed that the child's infected lung required *oral* antibiotics and not continued *intravenous* treatments, she argued forcibly. After the child was discharged the situation escalated and a telephone call was made to the bacteriology laboratory with false information about the species of bacterium identified in the child's sputum. Then the mother made a telephone call to the local Cystic Fibrosis Foundation. Eventually the mother presented to the hospital the sputum of another child who was suffering from genuine cystic fibrosis. The mother was clearly informed by the doctors that 'it seemed that her child probably did not have cystic fibrosis, but because of the great pressures on her from having a sick child without a certain diagnosis, she seemed to need to have that label'.

With an escalating situation, and the risks to the child more in evidence, the child was placed temporarily under a legal order restricting visits by the parents. The father had remained rather distant throughout. In hospital, with this protection, the child ceased to vomit, gained weight dramatically and became more active and social. The child was subsequently placed with his grandparents for six months and then, contrary to medical advice, returned to his parents. The family did not attend for follow-up and the physicians expressed great concern about the child's ongoing welfare.

This last situation illustrates the presence of fabrication in the presence of an existing physical disorder. The observation of the child's subsequent thriving indicated an initial failure to thrive, which appeared to be at least in part due to active withholding of food, as well as other factors. Emesis (vomiting) also had been induced by the mother. The history had been life long.

Diabetes (Nading and Duval-Arnould, 1984)

A three-year-old girl had the signs and symptoms of diabetes mellitus fabricated by the mother. When the girl was presented at the clinic, her mother gave a three-week history of polydipsia (excessive drinking), polyuria (high output of urine), nocturnal enuresis (bed-wetting) and weight loss. The mother reported finding glucose 3+ on five measurements of her daughter's urine. Physical examination was normal, as was blood level of glucose and urine testing. In hospital the child had several fasting blood samples taken and the glucose level was normal on each of them. However, urine samples collected by her mother continued to show 2+ to 4+ glucose and small to large acetone (another indicator of likely diabetes). As a way of finding out if the mother was interfering with the urine samples, the child was given ascorbic acid in orange juice. From that time all samples collected by nurses contained the ascorbic acid and all samples collected by the mother did not, thus demonstrating that the mother was sourcing the urine from elsewhere.

Vomiting (McGuire and Feldman, 1989)

A three-year-old child was presented with intractable vomiting since infancy, which had resulted in multiple hospital admissions and eventually intravenous feeding. The mother frequently reported vomiting, which was never observed by others. One episode of 'vomiting blood' and tampering with the intravenous line was later discovered (presumably to obtain a sample of blood for the false report).

Illness induction

Illness induction by non-accidental poisoning (Rogers et al., 1976)

Six examples of non-accidental poisoning are reported. The first child, a baby of two months, was admitted to hospital on three occasions with a story presented by the mother of loss of appetite, difficulties breathing and dehydration. Investigation of the child's sodium (salt) and water handling revealed no abnormality. The mother's expressed breast milk was found to contain extraordinarily high sodium (salt) concentrations. Following introduction of a low-salt cow's milk feed the child remained well until a further admission. Then a similar episode occurred whilst on the ward. It was calculated that the mother had given the child 6 g (about 2.5 level teaspoons) of salt added to feeds over a 24-hour period.

The child returned to the hospital initially as an inpatient and later was seen weekly as an outpatient. The mother agreed to seek psychiatric help. The child was re-admitted twice over the next year with abscesses attributed by the mother to heel pricks and intra-muscular injections. At the age of one year the child was admitted moribund with evidence of salt poisoning.

A child of seven years was under the supervision of the hospital following the sudden death of his brother at the age of two years with hypernatraemia (a high level of salt in the blood) and sagittal sinus thrombosis after a prolonged illness with non-specific symptoms. From the age of four years the boy began to have attacks of sweating, dizziness and pallor for which no cause was found. At the age of seven years the boy was in a state of excessive dependence upon his mother and was socially with-drawn as a result of being subjected to severe over-protectiveness by her.

The child was admitted to the hospital curled up in a pushchair in which he had been staying day and night. The mother remained resident with the boy for five weeks and remained close by him. After discharge the attacks recurred and the elec-trolytes and electrocardiogram suggested poisoning by diuretics, which were found in his urine. The mother refused psychiatric help and the child remained in the care of the Local Authority.

The other four cases reported were: a two-year-old given barbiturates, a seven-year-old boy given Mandrax (also a bar-biturate), a girl of 15 months given dihydrocodeine (an opiate), a girl of two years given Phenformin (a medicine for diabetes which reduces blood sugar).

Administration of laxative medicine (Epstein et al., 1987)

An 18-month-old boy suffered from intractable diarrhoea. His mother had surreptitiously been feeding him with laxative medicines with a syringe, probably from the age of three months. It was noted that when the mother had returned to the family home for a few days the diarrhoea had ceased. Later the mother was observed using the syringe.

Smothering and recurrent apnoea (cessation of breathing) (Rosen, Frost and Glaze, 1986)

Eleven infants were noted to have suffered episodes of cessation of breathing, which required resuscitation, which began only in the presence of one parent and were subsequently witnessed by another adult. In two of these infants the mother was conclus-ively proven to have been smothering the child.

Skin rash (Jones, 1983)

A baby of $4\frac{1}{2}$ weeks was admitted to a specialist inpatient unit for two weeks' assessment after the health visitor and general prac-titioner noticed lesions (unusual marks) on her face. On exam-ination in hospital there were five discrete round, dug-out lesions, each of 4 mm diameter and surrounded by a rim of 1 mm wide of fibrotic, heaped-up scar tissue. The lesions were of different ages and were situated over the head and body. On two occasions lesions became active and bled during the admission, although they quickly recovered when securely covered. The mother attributed the lesions to a list of causes, which seemed to be highly unlikely. It was observed that the mother had similar lesions on the extensor surfaces of the forearms and lower legs. Clearly the mother had actually caused the lesions both on the child and herself. This is called 'dermatitis artefacta' by dermatologists.

Following psychological intervention, comprising supportive therapy with both parents and work with the mother in the nursery, the family were discharged from hospital. Although there was initial improvement, over six months single lesions continued to appear and later there was failure to thrive and rough handling of the child by the mother was observed by staff with the subsequent appearance of a bruise. At 18 months the parents began to row and five new lesions appeared on the face of the child. A Place of Safety Order was taken (this order was replaced by the Emergency Protection Order under the Children Act 1989) and then the child continued to live in long-term foster care, where she thrived.

Failure to thrive and deliberate withholding of food (Gray and Bentovim, 1996)

Ten examples were reported in which the parent withheld food deliberately and then presented the child for investigation as to why they were not thriving. A case is described to illustrate a typical presentation.

A boy of 23 months had been known to the hospital virtually since birth. During much of his life there had been considerable concern about his profound *failure to thrive* and developmental delay. The family seemed to be caring and providing a good standard of parenting, although there had been similar medical concerns about an older child. Intensive investigations had proved negative. The boy was admitted to the hospital, where his calorie intake was closely monitored. During a controlled study (undertaken by a dietician) a member of the ward team observed the mother secretly disposing of the child's food. Earlier it had been recorded, based on the mother's report, that the child had eaten all of the food, which had disappeared from his plate during the meal. The consultant had been puzzled as to why he was not thriving on that amount of calorie intake.

A possible fabricated psychiatric disorder (Fisher, Mitchell and Murdoch, 1993)

A 10-year-old boy was brought to the emergency room of a hospital by his 36-year-old mother who claimed a history of hallucinations, bizarre behaviour, and allergies. The boy had been fed on a strict vegetarian diet for the first four years of his life because of alleged multiple allergies. The mother had taken the boy to many doctors and had been dissatisfied with most opinions given. There was a series of difficulties from behaviour problems from age four, which increased and led to six months' foster care at age seven years. The boy had disclosed sexual abuse, which was confirmed, and he responded well to psychotherapy. The boy's mother was intensely over-involved with every aspect of his life and she insisted that allergies were the cause of all of his difficulties. Many agencies were involved.

The mother reported that the boy was experiencing hallucinations, although she insisted that he had total amnesia and only she could accurately report his experiences. Later it was revealed that the mother provided detailed descriptions to the boy of his 'symptoms'. Initially the boy was given a diagnosis of paranoid schizophrenia and treated with the medications for that serious mental illness. When the boy was seen for assessment by the authors of the paper he presented with a normal mental state. His mother, however, had an interesting and abnormal mental state, which was grandiose, suspicious, circumstantial and over-inclusive in her thinking. The boy was admitted to an inpatient psychiatric unit, taken off all medication and observed for six weeks during which time there was no evidence of a psychotic illness. The boy did indicate fears of victimization, rejection, abandonment and a poor self-image. There were few behavioural problems. However, when his mother visited he was oppositional and ignored his peers. There was no evidence of allergies when foods were re-introduced.

By contrast the mother was found to be initially anxious, agitated, aloof, and mistrustful. Following the building of a working relationship with members of staff it became possible to carry out several in-depth assessments of the mother's mental state. Fabrication of the child's symptoms and *symptom coaching* were suspected and child protective services became involved. The boy was discharged home under supervision from child protective services and the mother engaged in intensive psychotherapy.

The history included a suspected personal and family history of sexual abuse. There was an uncertain history of nursing training and an extensive eventful personal history was presented leading to a suspicion of 'pseudologia fantastica' (*see* Glossary). The mother demonstrated features of both Narcissistic and Histrionic personality disorders. After nine months of psychotherapy there were significant improvements, with a reduction of grandiosity, and she was no longer focusing on the children as problematic. In the mother her belief that her son's allergies were the cause of all of his problems had been almost given up.

Fabrication in the setting of genuine physical illness (Godding and Kruth, 1991)

In the setting of a children's asthma clinic the authors studied compliance with treatment and the possibility of poor management as a result of falsifying symptoms or manipulating treatment or investigations, or both. The authors identified 17 families from 1,648 asthmatic patients (approximately 1%) in which the management of the asthma was non-compliant for one or more of these reasons. Essentially two prominent features were that one of the parents had not been honest with the doctor and as a result of the mismanagement there was a harmful impact on the child's mental and physical well-being. As a result of the dishonesty 11 children in 10 families were significantly under-treated (a form of medical neglect) and seven children from seven families were over-treated (more typical of most examples of FII).

In the first group, despite the children being described by their parents as having severe asthma, either the prescribed treatments for acute asthma attacks were not given by the parents or ineffective treatments were given. In addition the preventative treatments were not given in five of the families. In these families at least one of the parents had suffered from a chronic medical condition in their own childhood, six of the ten mothers were clinically depressed and one was known to be abusing morphine. Five of the families refused to allow doctors to see their children.

In the second group the families appeared to behave 'as if they wanted their children to remain chronically ill'. All exaggerated descriptions of their child's illness, and some parents gave falsified accounts of symptoms. Six of the families over-used medications, for example giving oral corticosteriods or antibiotics for a common cold. Five of the seven mothers were clinically depressed and five of the families were always seeking medical advice.

Presentations in obstetric settings (Jureidini, 1993)

In one of the first papers on this subject Jureidini sets out to show:

- the importance of Factitious Disorder as a differential diagnosis in obstetrics
- its dangers to the foetus
- a clinically important link between obstetric complications (factitious and genuine) and FII.

The literature is briefly reviewed and six families in which the mother presented with Factitious Disorder in pregnancy (Obstetric Factitious Disorder) encountered in the author's practice are described. In these families six mothers were responsible for FII in 14 of their 19 children. For three mothers one or more pregnancies were complicated by significant obstetric events (a total of eight pregnancies). At least five mothers showed evidence of factitious behaviour during at least 13 of their pregnancies. The examples of subsequent FII included: apnoea with later glycerine poisoning (via an IV line), allegations of poisoning of two siblings, apnoea induced by asphyxiation, and fabricated epilepsy.

Combining the information from the literature review and the new cases reported by Jureidini, the most common presentations were antepartum haemorrhage and feigned premature labour.

The variety of presentations were: feigned rupture of membranes, induced postpartum bleeding leading to anaemia, self-induced vomiting presenting as hyperemesis gravidarum, false claims of reduced foetal movements, feigned pyrexia, feigned trophoblastic disease, and feigned seizures.

Symptom coaching

A question that may arise is that of 'collusion' by the child, i.e. how much is the child involved in the creation of the fabricated illness. Sanders (1995) addresses the phenomenon of *symptom coaching* in older children and describes a continuum of collusion: naivety (usually due to the young age of the child), passive acceptance, active participation, and active harm (when illness induction is involved). Sanders defines coaching as 'the invitation the parent may give to the child to participate in symptom production'. When the child appears to be actively involved in the process of fabrication the complexity of the situation increases and questions then arise concerning the possible motivations for the collusion with the carer. This is discussed in some detail by Sanders.

Examples of participation by the child

In both of the following examples the child participated in the creation of an impression of illness. In the first it is not clear whether the child verbally fabricated, or was experiencing symptoms of a psychological/psychiatric nature, although the impact on the child's life is severe. It is clear that the mother sought many medical opinions about the girl's problems. In the second example the child clearly actively fabricated. In the example already presented above described by Croft and Jervis (1989) the child of only four years actively participated in the deception.

Headaches (Woollcott et al., 1982)

A $13\frac{1}{2}$-year-old girl was referred to a child psychiatry service with a history of many absences from school; approximately 70 days per year over eight years. Complaints of daily frontero-temporal headache and diminished energy were of many years' duration. Medical examination and laboratory findings were normal. Over the previous five years the mother and child had consulted at least eight physicians on at least 20 occasions, and the patient had been hospitalised five times.

When at school the child functioned well academically, but had uncomfortable relationships with peers. The assessing psychiatrist considered that the relationship between the child and mother was pathologically close. The child's father was emotionally distant from the family. At follow-up the child remained in an overtly dependent attachment to her mother, reinforced by the belief that she was ill.

Urine infection (Sneed and Bell, 1976)

A 10-year-old boy was seen as a medical emergency because of intermittent, colic-like pains in the right abdomen for the previous 24 hours and passage of red blood in the urine the previous night. Examination and investigations were normal apart from the analysis of the urine, which demonstrated moderate occult blood, 6–8 red blood cells with shadow cells, rare white blood cells and a trace of protein. The child was seen by another medical team five days later and a fuller examination and investigations revealed no abnormalities. Notably a further urine sample was normal. The mother was advised to filter and screen the urine for stones if the symptoms recurred.

Three and a half months later the boy was re-presented with a history of a temperature, pains in the left flank and 'black specks' being passed in the urine. Examination revealed complaints of tenderness in the left costo-vertebral area (i.e. over the kidney). Urine showed positive for a slight amount of haemoglobin (a main component of blood cells). The black specks proved to be unidentifiable except for one, which appeared to be the leg of an insect. The child was treated with antibiotics and the need to collect passed stones was impressed on the mother and boy. The mother reported that the child had been feverish with colicky abdominal pains and had passed a stone via his penis. Over the next month he submitted several small stones, which, he claimed, had been passed over three episodes. It was learnt that he had been outdoors prior to the passage of the stones, which on examination were identified as small water-worn pebbles of quartz lightly stained with iron oxide.

A history emerged of recurrent absenteeism and truancy by the boy and his siblings, maternal hostility to the school authorities and a history of psychological difficulties in both parents. Following referral for psychological evaluation of the boy 12 months passed with no further medical presentations. The evaluation revealed a rather passive compliant person who had difficulty in expressing his needs in interpersonal relationships. There was an almost complete dependence on others, particularly his mother. It was also discovered that the boy had reported a series of illnesses and had sought and used numerous medical practitioners and facilities for treatment.

References

Croft RD, Jervis M. Munchausen's syndrome in a 4-year-old. *Archives of Disease in Childhood*. 1989; **64**: 740–1.

Epstein MA, Markowitz RL, Gallo DM, Holmes JW, Gryboski JD. Munchausen syndrome by proxy: considerations in diagnosis and confirmation by video surveillance. *Pediatrics*. 1987; **80**(2): 220–4.

Fisher GC, Mitchell I, Murdoch D. Munchausen's syndrome by proxy. The question of psychiatric illness in a child. *British Journal of Psychiatry*. 1993; **162**: 701–3.

Godding V, Kruth M. Compliance with treatment in asthma and Munchausen syndrome by proxy. *Archives of Disease in Childhood*. 1991; **66**: 956–60.

Gray J, Bentovim A. Illness induction syndrome: paper I – a series of 41 children from 37 families identified at the Great Ormond Street Hospital for Children NHS Trust. *Child Abuse and Neglect*. 1996; **20**: 655–73.

HM Government. *Safeguarding Children in Whom Illness is Fabricated or Induced*. London: Department for Education and Skills; 2007. www.everychildmatters. gov.uk/safeguarding

Jones DPH. Dermatitis artefacta in mother and baby as child abuse. *British Journal of Psychiatry*. 1983; **143**: 199–200.

Jureidini J. Obstetric Factitious Disorder and Munchausen syndrome by proxy. *Journal of Nervous and Mental Disease*. 1993; **181**: 135–7.

Lee DA. Munchausen syndrome by proxy in twins. *Archives of Disease in Childhood*. 1979; **54**(8): 646–7.

McGuire TL, Feldman KW. Psychologic morbidity of children subjected to Munchausen syndrome by proxy. *Pediatrics*. 1989; **83**(2): 289–92.

Nading JH, Duval-Arnould B. Factitious diabetes mellitus confirmed by ascorbic acid. *Archives of Disease in Childhood*. 1984; **59**(2): 166–7.

Orenstein DM, Wasserman AL. Munchausen syndrome by proxy simulating cystic fibrosis. *Pediatrics*. 1986; **78**(4): 621–4.

Rogers D, Tripp J, Bentovim A, Robinson A, Berry D, Goulding R. Non-accidental poisoning: an extended syndrome of child abuse. *British Medical Journal*. 1976; 1: 793–6.

Rosen CL, Frost JD, Glaze DG. Child abuse and recurrent infant apnea. *Journal of Pediatrics*. 1986; 109(6): 1065–7.

Roth D. How 'mild' is mild Munchausen syndrome by proxy? *Israel Journal of Psychiatry and Related Science*. 1990; 27: 160–7.

Sanders MJ. Symptom coaching: factitious disorder by proxy with older children. *Clinical Psychology Review*. 1995; 15: 423–42.

Sneed RC, Bell RF. The dauphin of Munchausen: factitious passage of renal stones in a child. *Pediatrics*. 1976; 58:127–30.

Stevenson RD, Alexander R. Munchausen syndrome by proxy presenting as a developmental disability. *Developmental and Behavioral Pediatrics*. 1990; 11: 262–4.

Warner JO, Hathaway MJ. The allergic form of Meadow's syndrome (Munchausen by proxy). *Archives of Disease in Childhood*. 1984; 59(2): 151–6.

Woollcott P, Aceto T, Rutt C, Bloom M, Glick R. Doctor shopping with the child as proxy patient: a variant of child abuse. *Journal of Pediatrics*. 1982; 101(2): 297–301.

Chapter 3

Impact on victims

Section headings
The short-term consequences for the victim
Mortality and serious physical effects
Co-morbidity in the short term
Effects at follow-up
Accounts by survivors
KEY WORDS/PHRASES
Mortality
Co-morbidity
Failure to thrive/faltering growth
Inappropriate medication
Neglect
Psychological morbidity
Follow-up studies

The short-term consequences for the victim

The cohort of children studied through the British Paediatric Surveillance Unit (BPSU) for the epidemiology study (described later in Chapter 8) were followed over a median of 24 months. The study is the largest carried out in the UK, and as far as we are aware in the world.

From 128 index cases it was possible to obtain data at follow-up for 119 children. Forty-six of the children were at home (with the abuser). Four of the 32 suffocation victims had died (one of whom had also been poisoned). Five of the 44 victims of non-accidental poisoning had died. Paediatricians reported that 27/111 of the original index children (24%) were still experiencing symptoms or signs as a direct consequence of the original abuse. Seventeen had behavioural problems, 10 physical problems and 13 (12%) were disabled. With regard to registration on a child protection register 108/120 children had been registered at the initial case conference; this had fallen significantly to 32% at the time of follow-up.

The occurrence of further abuse was investigated. Five children (of 30/39 at home at follow-up) who had suffered from fabrications, and had not been directly physically harmed as a result of the fabrications, were re-abused. In two cases this was further fabrication and in three emotional abuse. Nine children who had suffered from fabrication that had included direct physical abuse were returned home and one of these was re-abused. In addition, one of three children who had been suffocated and returned home was physically abused at follow-up.

Mortality and serious physical effects

The physical risks to the child victims of illness induction are perhaps evident from the descriptions above. There is published evidence that a small number of children die as a result and that others suffer from permanent physical effects. In the first comprehensive review of the literature Rosenberg (1987) reported that 10 children died of the 117 index children and also 10 of their siblings. The causes of death for the 10 index children was suffocation (4), salt poisoning (3), other poisoning (2), and uncertain (1). In a further comprehensive review, which excluded cases included by Rosenberg, Sheridan (2003) reported that there had been 27 deaths from the 451 cases reported in the literature. Again fabricated and induced apnoea was the single most common presentation of the deceased victims.

In addition, Sheridan (2003) reported that 33 victims had suffered from long-term, or permanent, disability. This may result from the method of illness induction and also from intrusive medical procedures (particularly if surgery is undertaken). One of the victims reported by Bools *et al.* (1992) suffered from quadriplegia and learning disability.

Co-morbidity in the short term

In addition to the index fabrication – the fabrication that was identified and led to protective action being taken by professionals – it has been reported that victims of FII have an increased likelihood of suffering from other difficulties and forms of maltreatment.

As part of a study of 56 families in which FII had occurred, other difficulties and forms of maltreatment (referred to as co-morbidity) suffered by the child victims and their siblings were examined and reported (Bools *et al.*, 1992). There were data for 54 living index children and 82 of 103 siblings.

Of the index children, 64% had been the victims of other fabrications in addition to the index fabrications. Twenty-nine per cent of the index children had a history of failure to thrive and 29% a history including non-accidental injury or inappropriate medication or neglect. Overall 73% of the index children had been affected by at least one of these additional problems.

Of the siblings 39% themselves had had illnesses fabricated by their mothers, and 17% had been affected by either failure to thrive, non-accidental injury, inappropriate medication or neglect.

Thus some of the other risks to children who are victims of FII include:

- failure to thrive
- non-accidental injury
- inappropriate medication and
- forms of neglect
- plus similar risks also apply to siblings.

Effects at follow-up

A follow-up of children from 56 families

The group of index children, and many of their siblings, reported above in the study of co-morbidity were followed up for 1 to 14 years (mean 5.6 years) (Bools *et al.*, 1993). The main findings were that 30 index children were living in families that included their biological mothers, whilst 24 were living with other family members or in substitute families. The researchers identified 10 examples of further fabrications during the follow-up period and 'other concerns' for a further eight children.

With regard to the development of the index children a range of difficulties were identified in 27 children, of whom 13 were residing with their mother and 14 elsewhere at the time of the study. The difficulties were conduct and emotional disorders, and problems related to school – the latter comprising problems in attention and concentration, and non-attendance.

In the opinion of the researchers the outcome for 20 of the index children (49% of those with sufficient data) was considered to be unacceptable.

A notable section of the paper summarized below draws attention to features associated with children who had better outcomes:

- continuous positive input from the father for three children (and additionally the paternal grandparents for two of these)
- successful short-term fostering before return to the mother for five children
- a long-term therapeutic relationship between the mother and a social worker for three mothers
- successful remarriage for two mothers
- early adoption for three children
- long-term placement with the same foster parents for one child.

Psychological morbidity (McGuire and Feldman, 1989)

The psychological morbidity of six child victims of FII is described in some detail by McGuire and Feldman from Seattle, USA (1989). The fabrications included illness induction by poisoning in two cases (with Ipecac: a laxative, and with Theophylline: a treatment for asthma). The latter was believed to be self-poisoning by the girl. The first child at 2.5 months was found difficult to feed by nursing staff. The mother's care of her had been observed to be 'mechanical'. When separated from her mother at the age of 10 months the girl developed physically and in her social interactions. The second child at the age of three years was observed to display a high level of activity on the ward, frequent temper tantrums, and aggression against staff, mother and other children. At the same time she was remarkably passive during medical examinations and compliant with her treatments. The younger brother of patient 2 was also the victim of fabrication and probable illness induction. He was observed to be a wary, wide-eyed child. He was agitated and fussy when fed by his mother, was difficult for staff to feed and then began to refuse to eat. He was observed to smile responsively for staff, but turn away from his mother.

A fourth child suffered from many fabrications, including eventually administration of honey to cause a false positive in a glucose tolerance test (for diabetes). The boy was placed in foster care. In a day programme for pre-school children with behaviour problems he was aggressive and angry. As he began to feel safe in foster care he felt able to describe force-feeding by his mother and beatings by his father. A fifth child, a girl of 13 years, suffered a seizure as a result of Theophylline toxicity. The girl by this age had developed a pattern of fabricating accounts of illness together with her mother. Whilst the girl was admitted to hospital she developed a conversion disorder manifested by an apparent paralysis of her left arm and leg. Symptoms resolved with physiotherapy, occupational and psychotherapy. The authors thought that the girl had taken the Theophylline in order to validate her contention that she was ill. A sixth child, the younger brother of the 13-year-old girl, was evaluated for sudden onset of apparent blindness and ataxia (instability of gait). All investigations including CT scan were normal. There was a long history of the mother presenting the boy with multiple complaints and spurious symptoms. The present disorder was thought to be a conversion disorder. The boy talked about his mother's partner returning home drunk and being abusive to the mother and children. The boy's symptoms (of the conversion disorder) recovered after a few sessions of therapy.

In these six examples McGuire and Feldman observe that the mothers had not allowed the children to separate and individuate from them, and the children had learnt to passively tolerate medical procedures. The older children had developed somatizing disorders in the form of serious conversion disorders (the presentation of physical symptoms in the absence of a physical causation).

In summary, the children presented with a variety of psychological (emotional) difficulties, depending on the age of the child, ranging from feeding problems in a young child to hysterical and behavioural problems in adolescence. The main caution of the paper is that, even with protection from continuing FII, the family environment is at risk of continuing to pose a significant psychological threat to the child over the medium and long term. The implication is that the family problems associated with the fabrication will need to be addressed, in addition to focusing on the behaviours and psychopathology of the perpetrator.

Papers summarizing published reports

Rosenberg summarized the literature available at the time of writing, in 1987, and concluded that long-term morbidity was 8% – a variety of physical, intellectual and psychological sequelae. In this author's opinion it is unlikely that long-term morbidity reported in the literature is, in the majority of cases, truly 'long term'. This is because most accounts are of a relatively short period of time during which the fabrication was recognized and appropriate action taken. In addition, the assessment of long-term morbidity also needs to consider the psychological sequelae in some depth, to take into account the effects of emotional abuse on the emotional and personality development of the children. For these reasons a summary of the many reports of morbidity in the many individual case reports in the literature is not presented here.

All of the follow-through studies have indicated the importance of medium-term or long-term safeguarding (protective) measures, if the child remains in the family of origin. How this may be achieved is addressed in the following chapters. It is perhaps useful to consider the impact of FII in the context of the more rigorous studies that have reported on follow-up of children who had suffered from physical abuse unconnected with FII. References to two such studies are provided in *further reading* below.

Accounts by survivors

An account written by a survivor and her therapist (Bryk and Siegel, 1997)

In a courageous account of her own abuse as a victim of FII, Mary Bryk, together with Patricia Siegel, provides a story from the inside. By combining the medical history from original case notes and through discussions between the victim and her therapist, the article chronicles eight years of the actual experiences with details of the long-term consequences on emotional and physical development, the factors that influence recovery and the impact on family relationships. The account is reproduced here.

The girl's first problems occurred at the age of two years following a trivial 'injury' to the right ankle that did not heal. Then followed eight years of infections of bone, which never fully healed. At the age of four years the right femur fractured whilst the girl was in hospital. Severe problems continued for years, suspected to be infections. At age six years the right arm became problematic in a similar sequence. The initial injury and subsequent re-injuries were in fact as a result of repeated hammer blows made by the mother. The mother had deliberately introduced infections into open wounds. On one occasion the mother poured boiling water into an incision on the right arm.

This abuse ceased when, at the age of 10, the girl stood up to her mother and threatened to inform the doctor and teacher what had been happening to her. From that point the mother began to abuse the brother in a similar manner. The youngest sister and the father continued throughout not to believe what was happening to the two children. The girl had suffered a childhood of pain and lost time spent in hospital; the physical result was a right arm that was deformed, scarred and missing muscle mass, both legs were multiply scarred and asymmetrical and the right leg had loss of tissue. Psychologically the effects were also profound. Initially there was fear and anxiety that the physical abuse would resume. Following success at school contrary to the expectation and advice of the parents the girl left home to attend college at the age of 18 and returned home infrequently. After graduation the girl remained away from home and met her future husband at the age of 25. At the age of 30 after having two daughters the victim began psychological therapy. This was a combination of individual and group therapy. It helped to know that the abuse suffered had been given a name. For the first time what had happened throughout childhood was talked about. There was psychological recovery. There was no further contact with the parents.

A book written by a survivor

A personal account of living through a childhood as victim of fabricated and induced illness is presented in detail in the recent book *Sickened* written by the child victim when she reached adulthood (Gregory, 2004). The book details a childhood of being subjected to medical investigations, medication and procedures including surgery. Life began as a low-birth-weight baby; a product of her mother's self-starved and eventually anaemic body. The father was unassertive and apparently uninterested in the illnesses created by his wife for their daughter. The main symptoms reported by the mother eventually suggested heart disease in the child. From early years the mother coached the child to behave in a sick way in preparation for visits to the doctor. The accounts of the changeable psychological state of the mother and other examples of deception that she carried out provide a vivid account of widely disturbed psychological functioning. The accounts of the mother's own childhood and teenage years provide some understanding of how the behaviour patterns developed in response to serious emotional adversities, including exploitative abuse. The book charts the development of the alternative view of herself gradually formed by the child victim. Escape from the situation, in the absence of a responsible adult who might have helped, followed years of unchallenged presentations to various doctors. The author tried to balance maintaining a relationship with her mother with escape from the role of sick victim. In the end this proved virtually impossible and upon return to the remarried mother's home the author realizes that the mother has been fabricating illness in her much younger half-sister.

References

Bools CN, Neale BA, Meadow SR. Co-morbidity associated with fabricated illness (Munchausen syndrome by proxy). *Archives of Disease in Childhood.* 1992; **67**: 77–9.

Bools CN, Neale BA, Meadow SR. Follow up of victims of fabricated illness (Munchausen Syndrome by Proxy). *Archives of Disease in Childhood.* 1993; **69**: 625–30.

Bryk M, Siegel PT. My mother caused my illness: the story of a survivor of Munchausen by Proxy Syndrome. *Pediatrics.* 1997; **100**: 1–7.

Davis P, McClure RJ, Rolfe K, Chessman N, Pearson S, Sibert JR, Meadow R. Procedures, placement, and risks of further abuse after Munchausen Syndrome by Proxy, non-accidental poisoning and non-accidental suffocation. *Archives of Disease in Childhood.* 1998; **78**: 217–21.

Gregory J. *Sickened. The true story of a lost childhood.* London: Arrow Books; 2004.

McGuire TL, Feldman KW. Psychologic morbidity of children subjected to Munchausen syndrome by proxy. *Pediatrics.* 1989; **83**(2): 289–92.

Rosenberg DA. Web of deceit: a literature review of Munchausen syndrome by proxy. *Child Abuse and Neglect.* 1987; 11(4): 547–63.

Sheridan MS. The deceit continues; an updated literature review of Munchausen Syndrome by Proxy. *Child Abuse and Neglect.* 2003; 27(4): 431–51.

Further reading

Gibbons J, Gallagher B, Bell C, Gordon D. *Development after Physical Abuse in Early Childhood.* London: HMSO; 1995.

Lynch MA, Roberts J. *Consequences of Child Abuse.* London: Academic Press; 1982.

Chapter 4

Behaviour, relationships and psychopathology

Section headings
Behaviour of fabricators
The mother–child relationship
Psychopathology
Overview of psychopathology
Fathers as fabricators
KEY WORDS/PHRASES
Parent over-involvement
Over-dependent
Psychopathology
Somatizing disorders
Somatoform Disorder
Factitious Disorder
Munchausen Syndrome
Personality disorder
Psychological defences

Behaviour of fabricators

Behaviour with the child in hospital

The most common behaviour reported in many examples in the literature is of a fabricating parent who appears to be caring and over-involved in the care of her child in hospital. Many workers have reported observations of a mother who rarely leaves her child's side whilst on the paediatric ward (Chan *et al.*, 1986; Epstein *et al.*, 1987; Fleisher and Ament, 1977; Koch and Hoiby, 1988; Malatack *et al.*, 1985; Miller, 1987; Nicol and Eccles, 1985; Pickford *et al.*, 1988; Rosen *et al.*, 1983; Warner and Hathaway, 1984). In addition, the mother reported by Wood *et al.* (1989) was noted to be reluctant to give up vital sign monitoring and administering prescribed medication to her child.

Maintenance of close proximity may facilitate direct manipulation of the physical state of the child by controlling food intake or by giving medicines, prescribed or otherwise, whilst the child is an inpatient. Rosen *et al.* (1983) reported that an apparent strong loving bond between mother and baby had been noted over a period when the mother was intermittently smothering the baby whilst on the ward.

The picture of a caring mother, who is close to her child, albeit unusually close, may be considered the 'classical' behaviour of the parent in FII. This is not, however, the only picture that has been reported. Sometimes the mother did not remain on the ward with the child and on occasions staff had voiced their concerns about the quality of care given to the child or the relationship between mother and child (Gray and Bentovim, 1996; Koch and Hoiby, 1988; Nicol and Eccles, 1985; Pickford *et al.*, 1988; Warner and Hathaway, 1984). Nicol and Eccles (1985) described a mother as cold and aloof, and Koch and Hoiby (1988) as displaying frank negative feelings towards the boy.

Behaviour with hospital staff

It has been reported on a number of occasions that parents were very sociable whilst on the ward, forming close relationships with nurses and junior medical staff, and also with other resident parents (Epstein *et al.*, 1987; Guandolo, 1985; Krener and Adelman, 1988; Meadow, 1982; Miller, 1987; Pickford *et al.*, 1988; Rosen *et al.*, 1983). Some mothers who fabricated illness had been noted to be surprisingly calm and trusting of the doctors despite the seriousness of their child's condition (Miller, 1987). The comfortableness of being (often living) in the hospital environment, and in the interactions with the healthcare staff, sometimes have led to quite close relationships being formed, thus adding greatly to the disbelief of the staff when the possibility of fabrication is first considered. The behaviour of the staff, having not even considered fabrication as a cause of the child's illness, may continue to reinforce the fabricator's view of the child as actually being ill.

Other mothers, however, were highly critical of the doctors (Warner and Hathaway, 1984; Woollcott *et al.*, 1982). Masterson *et al.* (1988) describe how an initial good rapport between doctor and mother changed into conflict with staff as organic causes for the illness were eliminated. The mother reported by Pickford *et al.* (1988) was anxious rather than calm.

The mother–child relationship

Accompanying the frequent observation that in 'classical FII' the mother remains unusually close (geographically) to her child is the notion that the mother is psychologically over-involved with, and over-dependent on, her child. Waller (1983) referred to this as 'the rather startling tie that exists between parent and child'. In the account given by a mother described by Pickford *et al.* (1988) the mother talked about her, and her husband, having the children to create a world that neither she nor her husband had experienced. The authors commented that the mother had poor self-boundaries and used the children as self-objects.

When a mother, already suffering from a somatizing disorder herself, also has a disturbed psychological boundary with her child it is possible to view FII, at least in part, as a 'spill over' phenomenon of the mother's own somatizing. This seems a reasonable way of viewing the situation when the child's illness is similar to that of the mother. Warner and Hathaway (1984), writing about factitious allergy affecting 17 children, noted that five (of the 11) mothers were on diets themselves without any obvious justification. A mother with an eating disorder poisoned her child with Ipecac producing diarrhoea and failure to thrive (Feldman *et al.*, 1989). Mothers described by Jones (1983) and by Stankler (1977) both produced skin lesions (dermatitis artefacta) in themselves and their children.

The desire of the mother to see the child as being ill may be strong. Warner and Hathaway (1984) commented that 'the parental obsession with diagnosis was very abnormal'. A mother who carried out a sophisticated fabrication of cystic fibrosis in her child was seen by a psychiatrist who concluded that:

> *the mother seems to be obsessed with a diagnosis being made on her son and that that diagnosis be cystic fibrosis. She appears to be obsessed to the point that she would fabricate information with the irrational belief that her son would have a better chance of being treated and cured should the diagnosis, even an inappropriate one, be made. (Orenstein and Wasserman, 1986)*

The mother described by Pickford *et al.* (1988) who had fabricated a series of illnesses demonstrated over-valued ideas (defined by

Simms, 1988, as 'an acceptable, comprehensible idea pursued by the patient beyond the bounds of reason') about her own and her children's bodies. The four mothers described by Woollcott *et al.* (1982) exhibited paranoid thinking and a conviction of serious medical illness in their child which approached delusional proportions.

Psychopathology

The significance of the somatizing disorder

There have been very many reports of 'somatizing disorders' in fabricating mothers (Ackerman and Strobel, 1981; Black, 1981; Bourchier, 1983; Epstein *et al.*, 1987; Fleisher and Ament, 1977; Geelhoed and Pemberton, 1985; Griffith, 1988; Hodge *et al.*, 1982; Lee, 1979; Livingston, 1987; Mehl *et al.*, 1990; Outwater *et al.*, 1981; Palmer and Yoshimura, 1984; Pickford *et al.*, 1988; Richardson, 1987; Samuels *et al.*, 1992; Stankler, 1977; Verity *et al.*, 1979; Wood *et al.*, 1989; Woollcott *et al.*, 1982). As part of the study of 56 families (Bools *et al.*, 1994) previously referred to in Chapter 3, it proved possible to report on the lifetime history of 47 mothers who had fabricated or induced illness in their child. Thirty-four of the mothers had a history of a somatizing disorder (a Factitious Disorder or a Somatoform Disorder). In a sub-group who had been interviewed it was of interest that in three cases the somatizing had commenced before school-leaving age and had been linked with school non-attendance. In at least 10 of the cases the disorders had been of chronic duration.

Livingston (1987) reports in detail on two mothers who fabricated and both were diagnosed with **Somatization Disorder** (*see* DSM disorders in the Appendix). The diagnoses were based on semi-structured interviews of three hours and examination of all available records.

The first woman had been poisoning her child with Ipecac (a laxative), Nortriptyline and Protriptyline (both antidepressants). An investigation revealed that three infants had been placed with her for adoption and two of them had died. The third child was placed elsewhere after being admitted to hospital with blood in the nappy, which was proven to have come from the mother.

The woman had an extensive medical and psychiatric history. From her early thirties she had been treated by four psychiatrists for symptoms of depression, anxiety, marital problems and drug dependence. From her early twenties she had been admitted to hospital 20 times for a variety of symptoms and had had surgery on at least four occasions, including a hysterectomy and two laminectomies. The woman had 21 additional medically unexplained symptoms for which she had sought treatment. The background included the suicide of her father under a cloud of suspicion about his honesty. She had completed one year of nursing school but was dismissed as 'unsuitable'. The history and examination did not reveal further evidence of other psychiatric conditions.

A 28-year-old mother was found to be poisoning her three-year-old daughter with Phenobarbitol. The child had been admitted to hospital on a total of 12 occasions, in four different hospitals. The mother herself had been in hospital at least 15 times since the age of 12. Perhaps notably on one occasion during her first year of nursing training she was hospitalized for suspected meningitis and had not returned to the course. The woman had presented with 18 other complaints for which she had seen a doctor; these included headaches, paraesthesias, hearing loss, blurred vision, weight fluctuations, nausea, vomiting throughout pregnancy, chest pains and dyspareunia. No organic cause was found to account for these symptoms. When a doctor had suggested a psychological basis, she had not returned to that doctor. The background was unremarkable, although her father was a 'reformed alcoholic'. The woman described herself as an 'extrovert' and was described by the author to be somewhat flamboyant in dress and manner. There was no evidence of other psychiatric disorders.

Livingston concludes that both subjects met the criteria for DSM-III *Somatization Disorder*, which was considered to be compatible with the reports of Hysterical and Borderline personality diagnoses reported by others. There was no evidence that their own symptoms had been voluntarily produced and therefore they did not meet the criteria for *Factitious Disorder*.

Self-harm and addictive behaviours

A history of self-harm by drug overdose has been reported by other authors (Alexander *et al.*, 1990; Fialkov, 1984; Fleisher and Ament, 1977; Griffith, 1988; Hosch, 1987; Palmer and Yoshimura, 1984). In addition, eight of the 13 mothers reported by Samuels *et al.* (1992) had a history of self-harm, six by overdose. Alcohol dependence has been reported (Black, 1981; Stankler, 1977) and the mother reported by Dershewitz *et al.* (1976) suffered from both alcohol and heroin addiction.

Twenty-six of 56 fabricating mothers (Bools *et al.*, 1994) had a history of some form of self-harm and 10 of addictive behaviours (alcohol or substance misuse – including prescribed medication).

Eating disorders

A number of fabricating mothers have been reported to suffer from an eating disorder. The mother reported by Feldman *et al.* (1989) expressed the wish that her children should not become fat and gave them Ipecac (a laxative) to cause *failure to thrive*. The mother suffered from a serious eating disorder herself. Samuels *et al.* (1992) noted that 10 of the mothers had suffered from an eating disorder; five from anorexia and weight loss, and five had been grossly overweight. The mother reported by White *et al.* (1985) was noted to be withdrawn, lacked motivation and was anorexic with weight loss.

Psychosis and depression

There have been very few examples of FII associated with a psychotic illness. One of the mothers described by Warner and Hathaway (1984), who treated her daughter as if she had very serious allergies, eventually had a 'nervous breakdown' which was diagnosed as schizophrenia. One of the mothers described by Woollcott *et al.* (1982) had a previous diagnosis of schizophrenia combined with multiple somatizations, although it is not clear whether the mother was actively ill with schizophrenia at the time of the fabrications. The mother described by Stone (1989) had received a diagnosis of chronic paranoid schizophrenia. Rogers *et al.* (1976) described a mother who had a severe depressive illness with retardation and depersonalization. The mother reported by Hosch (1987) suffered from 'severe depression'. A number of workers have reported that the mothers suffered from varieties of depression (Ackerman and Strobel, 1981; Epstein *et al.*, 1987; Kravitz and Wilmott, 1990; McGuire and Feldman, 1989), depression with character disorder (Watson *et al.*, 1979), or depression with personality disorder (Fialkov, 1984; Stevenson and Alexander, 1990).

Antisocial behaviour

Authors have noted the presence of other antisocial behaviour displayed by fabricating mothers. Alexander *et al.* (1990) noted that there had been four fires in the home of a mother who poisoned her child with arsenic, strongly suggesting arson. The mother reported by Epstein *et al.* (1987), who worked as a nurse's aid, had been dismissed for stealing medication from patients on a number of occasions. The mother reported by Jones *et al.* (1986) robbed the person she was staying with. One of the mothers described by Samuels *et al.* (1992), when she was 17 years old and together with her sister, had abducted a baby. Both had been placed on probation. Nine of the 56 women (Bools *et al.*, 1994) had a forensic history, which was independent of convictions related to child abuse. The offences included four of arson.

Personality disorder

Many authors have reported the features of various personality disorders in perpetrators of MSP: *Borderline* features (Atoynatan *et al.*, 1988; Chan *et al.*, 1986; Epstein *et al.*, 1987; Griffith, 1988; Hodge *et al.*, 1982; Pickford *et al.*, 1988), *Histrionic/Hysterical* features (Black, 1981; Epstein *et al.*, 1987; Fialkov, 1984; Fisher *et al.*, 1993; Griffith, 1988; Stankler, 1977; Stevenson and Alexander, 1990), and *Narcissistic* features (Chan *et al.*, 1986; Fisher *et al.*, 1993; Griffith, 1988; Rosen *et al.*, 1983) have all been described. Following assessment using a standard interview to assess the presence of personality disorders, Bools *et al.* (1994) identified the most common features as *Histrionic* and *Borderline*, with *Antisocial* and *Avoidant* features being the next most common. Seventeen of the 19 women interviewed received a diagnosis of a Personality Disorder.

Overview of psychopathology

Whilst the features referred to in the above paragraphs are commonly reported in fabricators of FII in children it is critically important to appreciate that such features *may not be present*. Published accounts probably report on more extreme examples of FII which include features of the fabricators. Thus there is *no single 'profile'* of behaviour, of personality or of psychiatric disorders in fabricators.

Fathers as fabricators

There are a small number of reports of the father of the child fabricating illness or perpetrating the induction of illness. Dine and McGovern (1982) reported a father who poisoned his seven-month-old son with Glutethimide. The father was a physician and subsequently committed suicide. Osborne (1976) reported a father who was himself epileptic and took Phenobarbitone and Phenytoin. The child was poisoned with the barbiturate and another unidentified drug. The father also admitted administering the medication to two older siblings.

Makar and Squier (1990) reported a father who smothered his baby and was observed by a nurse to be doing so. The mother was not present at the time. The typical history of apnoea had been given and investigations carried out. The father also stated that he had seen bright red blood in the child's stool. Morris (1985) reported a baby boy who was smothered by his father. After being observed the father (aged 18) admitted the smothering and previous similar episodes which had led to cyanosis. Once again the mother was not involved. The father had a history of being abused as a child, although the details were not given. Father and mother had a chaotic lifestyle with little social support.

In the report by Zohar et al. (1987) the father presented his five-year-old son with recurrent external otitis (an infection of the outer part of the ear). When the child was examined chalk was found in the ear on three occasions. The father was then recognised as being a former patient of the ENT department previously treated for what was almost certainly a somatizing disorder, most likely a factitious disorder, of the sinuses. The father left angrily when he learnt of the suspicion of the staff so no further information was given.

In the account of 37 families who had presented at Great Ormond Street Hospital for Children reported by Gray and Bentovim (1996) in three cases the father had been responsible for the induction of illness. In one of these the illness was induced by the administration of salt.

References

Ackerman NB, Strobel CT. Polle syndrome: chronic diarrhea in Munchausen's child. *Gastroenterology*. 1981; 81(6): 1140–2.

Alexander R, Smith W, Stevenson R. Serial Munchausen syndrome by proxy. *Pediatrics*. 1990; 86(4): 581–5.

American Psychiatric Association. *Diagnostic and Statistical Manual for Mental Disorders (Fourth Edition)*. Washington DC: American Psychiatric Association; 1994.

Atoynatan TH, O'Reilly E, Loin L. Munchausen syndrome by proxy. *Child Psychiatry and Human Development*. 1988; 19(1): 3–13.

Black D. The extended Munchausen syndrome: a family case. *British Journal of Psychiatry*. 1981; 138: 466–9.

Bools CN, Neale BA, Meadow SR. Munchausen Syndrome by Proxy: a study of psychopathology. *Child Abuse and Neglect*. 1994; 18: 773–88.

Bourchier D. Bleeding ears: case report of Munchausen syndrome by proxy. *Australian Paediatric Journal*. 1983; 19(4): 256–7.

Chan DA, Salcedo JR, Atkins DM, Ruley EJ. Munchausen syndrome by proxy: a review and case study. *Journal of Pediatric Psychology*. 1986; 11(1): 71–80.

Dershewitz R, Vestal B, Maclaren NK, Cornblath M. Transient hepatomegaly and hypoglycemia: a consequence of malicious insulin administration. *American Journal of Diseases of Children*. 1976; 130: 998–9.

Dine MS, McGovern ME. Intentional poisoning of children – an overlooked category of child abuse: report of seven cases and review of the literature. *Pediatrics*. 1982; 70(1): 32–5.

Epstein MA, Markowitz RL, Gallo DM, Holmes JW, Gryboski JD. Munchausen syndrome by proxy: considerations in diagnosis and confirmation by video surveillance. *Pediatrics*. 1987; 80(2): 220–4.

Feldman KW, Christopher DM, Opheim KB. Munchausen syndrome/bulimia by proxy: ipecac as a toxin in child abuse. *Child Abuse and Neglect*. 1989; 13: 257–61.

Fialkov MJ. Peregrination in the problem pediatric patient: the pediatric Munchhausen syndrome? *Clinical Pediatrics*. 1984; 23(10): 571–5.

Fisher GC, Mitchell I, Murdoch D. Munchausen's syndrome by proxy. The question of psychiatric illness in a child. *British Journal of Psychiatry*. 1993; 162: 701–3.

Fleisher D, Ament ME. Diarrhea, red diapers, and child abuse. *Clinical Pediatrics.* 1977; **17**(9): 820–4.

Geelhoed GC, Pemberton PJ. SIDS, seizures or 'sophageal reflux? Another manifestation of Munchausen syndrome by proxy. *Medical Journal of Australia.* 1985; **143**(8): 357–8.

Gray J, Bentovim A. Illness induction syndrome: paper I – a series of 41 children from 37 families identified at the Great Ormond Street Hospital for Children NHS Trust. *Child Abuse and Neglect.* 1996; **20**: 655–73.

Griffith JL. The family systems of Munchausen syndrome by proxy. *Family Process.* 1988; **27**: 423–37.

Guandolo VL. Munchausen syndrome by proxy: an outpatient challenge. *Pediatrics.* 1985; **75**(3): 526–30.

Hodge D, Schwartz W, Sargent J, Bodurtha J, Starr S. The bacteriologically battered baby: another case of Munchausen syndrome by proxy. *Annals of Emergency Medicine.* 1982; **11**(4): 205–7.

Hosch IA. Munchausen syndrome by proxy. *American Journal of Maternal Child Nursing.* 1987; **12**(1): 48–52.

Jones DPH. Dermatitis artefacta in mother and baby as child abuse. *British Journal of Psychiatry.* 1983; **143**: 199–200.

Jones JG, Butler HL, Hamilton B, Perdue JD, Stern HP, Woody RC. Munchausen syndrome by proxy. *Child Abuse and Neglect.* 1986; **10**: 33–40.

Koch C, Hoiby N. Severe child abuse presenting as polymicrobial bacteremia. *Acta Paediatrica Scandinavica.* 1988; **77**: 940–3.

Kravitz RM, Wilmott RW. Munchausen syndrome by proxy presenting as factitious apnea. *Clinical Pediatrics.* 1990; **29**: 587–92.

Krener P, Adelman R. Parent salvage and parent sabotage in the care of chronically ill children. *American Journal of Diseases of Children.* 1988; **142**(9): 945–51.

Lee DA. Munchausen syndrome by proxy in twins. *Archives of Disease in Childhood.* 1979; **54**(8): 646–7.

Livingston R. Maternal somatization disorder and Munchausen syndrome by proxy. *Psychosomatics.* 1987; **28**(4): 213–15.

Makar AF, Squier PJ. Munchausen syndrome by proxy: father as perpetrator. *Pediatrics.* 1990; **85**(3): 370–3.

Malatack JJ, Wiener ES, Gartner JC, Zitelli BJ, Brunetti E. Munchausen syndrome by proxy: a new complication of central venous catheterization. *Pediatrics.* 1985; **75**(3): 523–5.

Masterson J, Dunworth R, Williams N. Extreme illness exaggeration in pediatric patients: a variant of Munchausen's by proxy? *American Journal of Orthopsychiatry.* 1988; **58**(2): 188–95.

McGuire TL, Feldman KW. Psychologic morbidity of children subjected to Munchausen syndrome by proxy. *Pediatrics.* 1989; **83**(2): 289–92.

Meadow R. Munchausen syndrome by proxy. *Archives of Disease in Childhood.* 1982; **57**(2): 92–8.

Mehl AL, Coble L, Johnson S. Munchausen syndrome by proxy: A family affair. *Child Abuse and Neglect.* 1990; **14**: 577–85.

Miller S. Family court: matter of Jessica Z. *New York Law Journal.* 1987; **3 March**: 13.

Morris B. Child abuse manifested as factitious apnea. *Southern Medical Journal.* 1985; **78**: 1013–14.

Nicol AR, Eccles M. Psychotherapy for Munchausen syndrome by proxy. *Archives of Disease in Childhood.* 1985; **60**(4): 344–8.

Orenstein DM, Wasserman AL. Munchausen syndrome by proxy simulating cystic fibrosis. *Pediatrics.* 1986; **78**(4): 621–4.

Osborne JP. Non-accidental poisoning and child abuse. *British Medical Journal.* 1976; **May 15**: 1211.

Outwater KM, Lipnick RN, Luban NLC, Ravenscroft K, Ruley EJ. Factitious hematuria: diagnosis by minor blood group typing. *Journal of Pediatrics.* 1981; **98**(1): 95–7.

Palmer AJ, Yoshimura GJ. Munchausen syndrome by proxy. *J American Academy Child and Adolescent Psychiatry.* 1984; **23**(4): 503–8.

Pickford E, Buchanan N, McLaughlan S. Munchausen syndrome by proxy: a family anthology. *Medical Journal of Australia.* 1988; **148**(12): 646–50.

Richardson GF. Munchausen syndrome by proxy. *American Family Physician.* 1987; **36**(1): 119–23.

Rogers D, Tripp J, Bentovim A, Robinson A, Berry D, Goulding R. Non-accidental poisoning: an extended syndrome of child abuse. *British Medical Journal.* 1976; **1**: 793–6.

Rosen CL, Frost JD, Bricker T, Tarnow JD, Gillette PC, Dunlavy S. Two siblings with recurrent cardiorespiratory arrest: Munchausen syndrome by proxy or child abuse? *Pediatrics.* 1983; **71**(5): 715–20.

Samuels MP, McClaughlin W, Jacobson RR, Poets CF, Southall DP. Fourteen cases of imposed upper airway obstruction. *Archives of Disease in Childhood.* 1992; **67**: 162–70.

Simms A. *Symptoms in the Mind: an introduction to descriptive psychopathology.* London: Baillière Tindall; 1988.

Stankler L. Factitious skin lesions in a mother and two sons. *British Journal of Dermatology.* 1977; **97**: 217–19.

Stevenson RD, Alexander R. Munchausen syndrome by proxy presenting as a developmental disability. *Developmental and Behavioral Pediatrics.* 1990; **11**: 262–4.

Stone FB. Munchausen by proxy syndrome: An unusual form of child abuse. *Social Casework.* 1989; **April**: 243–6.

Verity CM, Winckworth C, Burman D, Stevens D, White RJ. Polle syndrome: children of Munchausen. *British Medical Journal.* 1979; **2**(6187): 422–3.

Waller DA. Obstacles to the treatment of Munchausen by proxy syndrome. *J American Academy Child and Adolescent Psychiatry.* 1983; **22**(1): 80–5.

Warner JO, Hathaway MJ. The allergic form of Meadow's syndrome (Munchausen by proxy). *Archives of Disease in Childhood.* 1984; **59**(2): 151–6.

Watson JBG, Davies JM, Hunter JLP. Non-accidental poisoning in childhood. *Archives of Disease in Childhood.* 1979; **54**(2): 143–4.

White ST, Voter K, Perry J. Surreptitious warfarin ingestion. *Child Abuse and Neglect.* 1985; **9**(3): 349–52.

Wood PR, Fowlkes J, Holden P, Casto D. Fever of unknown origin for six years: Munchausen syndrome by proxy (clinical conference). *Journal of Family Practice.* 1989; **28**: 391–5.

Woollcott P, Aceto T, Rutt C, Bloom M, Glick R. Doctor shopping with the child as proxy patient: a variant of child abuse. *Journal of Pediatrics*. 1982; 101(2): 297–301.

Zohar Y, Avidan G, Shvili Y, Laurian N. Otolaryngologic cases of Munchausen's syndrome. *Laryngoscope*. 1987; 97(2): 201–3.

Further reading

Bass C, Murphy M. Somatoform and personality disorders: syndromal co-morbidity and overlapping developmental pathways. *J Psychosomatic Research*. 1995; 39: 403–27.

Eisendrath SJ. Factitious illness: a clarification. *Psychosomatics*. 1984; 25: 110–17.

Falkov A. *Crossing Bridges. Training resources for working with mentally ill parents and their children. Reader – for managers, practitioners and trainers*. Brighton: Pavilion Publishing, for the Department of Health; 1998.

Chapter 5

Explanatory models: trying to understand FII

Section headings

Understanding using a developmental and family systems approach

A narrative approach

Early life experiences and family patterns of fabricators

Trans-generational attachment

Dimensions of parent behaviour

The psychosomatic continuum: what is not FII

The vulnerable child

Illness behaviour and abnormal illness behaviour

What is somatization?

What is Somatization Disorder?

What influences the development of somatization?

KEY WORDS/PHRASES

Parental perception that the child is ill

Ambivalence towards the child

Care by proxy

Narrative approach

Attention seeking

Abnormal care-giving behaviours

Abnormal care-eliciting behaviours

Internal working model

Psychosomatic continuum

Sick role

Somatization Disorder

Vulnerability

Vulnerable child syndrome

Understanding using a developmental and family systems approach

Based on their experience of the 41 examples of FII, Gray and Bentovim (1996) present an understanding of the processes leading to illness fabrication and induction using a developmental and family systems approach. This includes consideration of the attachment of the parent, usually the mother, to the child, in the context of the parents' own life experiences and takes into account that of the other partner. It is helpful for understanding the FII situation to consider processes **and also** descriptive terms, such as psychiatric diagnoses: the latter may be helpful for communication between professionals.

It appears that the (mis)perception that the child is ill, combined with the parent's ambivalence towards the child, becomes interwoven into a belief that the child is ill. This belief is confirmed by the medical response and in the cases described by Gray and Bentovim had resulted in the child being admitted to a tertiary care hospital for assessment and treatment. Here the parent received the care accorded to the parent of a sick child. The confirmation that the child could be ill served both to maintain the perception of the child as ill and to act as a solution to the parent's problems. Sometimes active induction was then necessary to maintain medical involvement with both the child in the sick role and the parent.

The high levels of early privations, and stressful and traumatic events experienced by the mothers (and some fathers) were considered to have played a role in the genesis of the relationship difficulties and Personality Disorders, and the ambivalent attitudes to the child (*see* Chapter 4). Somatization and the associated help seeking through medical referral had become an established, almost normal, frequent mode of seeking and receiving help. The histories of the children also contributed to the development of the FII. The histories were characterized by difficulties in conception or delivery, prematurity, failure to thrive and health concerns. Any one, or a combination, of these difficulties might provide a seed of an idea, which develops in the mind of the parent, that the child is basically unhealthy. What then happens probably depends on a combination of the established behaviour patterns of the parents combined with what is happening in the life of the parent, and affected by the response of the medical staff who are consulted. The nature of the questions asked by the medical staff and the investigations carried out can shape the responses by the parents. Professionals may then unwittingly share the parent's perception of the child's health and become a part of the solution to the family's problems.

The concerns of health professionals and the admission of the child to hospital result in the mother receiving the normal care and concern given to any mother who accompanies her child in hospital, thus providing *care by proxy* for the mother. One consequence is that concern is evoked in partners, extended family, and community members with one result that individual, marital and family problems were set aside and temporarily resolved by focusing on the sick child. In order to maintain this illusion the parent may need to continue the medical focus by inducing illness to keep a high level of concern by the medical staff on the child.

Elements of this process – the mechanisms underlying the process of illness induction – are shown in Figure 5.1, reproduced from Gray and Bentovim (1996).

A narrative approach

Loader and Kelly (1996) complement the approaches that focus on the characteristics of the mother and family in FII with a *narrative approach* which views FII as the outcome of a particular human story. They present a detailed history, linked with clinical and research findings, in an attempt to track the evolution of the fabricating behaviour. They suggest that FII is best seen as a process, and one in which the key relationship is between the mother and the child's doctor, which has important implications for the detection and management of the problem.

In order to fully appreciate the narrative around David (the victim of FII in this example) and his family, one really needs to read the paper in full. However, the key elements are presented here. Firstly here follows a brief account of the fabrication and management. At the age of five David had been admitted to hospital with a history of six reported 'fits'. Eventually after falling into a coma and requiring treatment in intensive care, David's urine was found to contain chloral hydrate (a sedative medication). After initial denial, the mother informed staff that she had given him the medication to calm him down, as his behaviour on the ward was an embarrassment to her. After two months in hospital David was discharged to foster care and after seven months returned home with supervision by social services under a continuing Care Order.

At this point the authors were contacted and agreed to carry out an assessment to advise in court proceedings as to whether the Care Order should be revoked. A very full history was taken of the child's development and the parent's view of the present

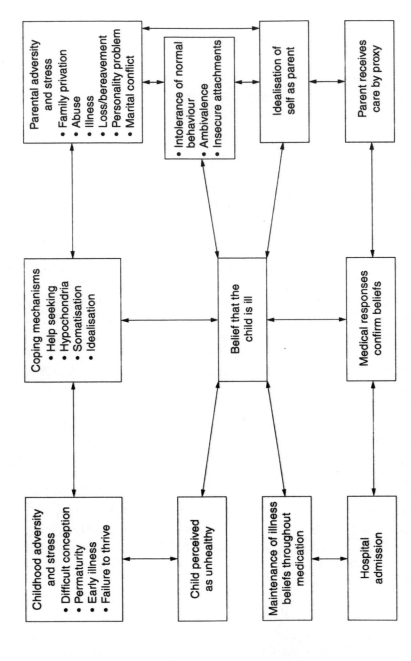

Figure 5.1 Mechanisms underlying the process of illness induction. From *JCAN* **20**(8): 655–73; 1996.

situation. David was seen at the family home and an assessment made of his psychological state and his view of the situation. The key points in the history follow. The family consisted of father (age 43) and mother (age 41); the index child David (age 8) had two brothers age 11 and 22 (living at home). In David's early life he had been investigated for milk intolerance and was given a special diet. From age three asthma was diagnosed and the 'blank episodes' were reported by mother. By age four the 'blank episodes' had developed into 'blackouts' and doctors thought David was suffering from epilepsy and therefore prescribed anti-convulsant medication. In order to try and help sleep problems the GP prescribed large amounts of chloral hydrate and another sedative. At school David was frequently drowsy; he was also sent to school strapped into a wheelchair and wearing a crash helmet.

The parents did not believe that the Care Order was necessary. The mother could not recall giving David the excessive medication although she 'knew that she did'. She suggested she must have been depressed. After David was removed from her care she had become severely depressed and sought psychiatric help although she declined to follow up the recommendation for individual psychotherapy. At the time of the assessment the mother saw David as a normal boy, although somewhat overactive and difficult to control. There had been problems at school with David telling incredible stories, which he maintained were true when confronted with absolute evidence that they were not true.

David was found to be immature, demanding, and confused about what had happened to him. It was interesting that he viewed the family's social worker as a friend and he wanted her to continue to come and see them: this was contrary to the view of his parents and brothers.

The authors examine the factors that may have contributed to the psychology and behaviour of the mother. The mother described a very unhappy childhood; in particular she had felt continually criticized by her mother, and paid little attention to by her father. After the FII was identified, the psychopathology had been assessed by a psychiatrist and no formal diagnosis was made. There had been a history of anorexia nervosa from age 14, and bouts of depression treated with medications and ECT, none of which had been found to be helpful. Although the mother had not grown up in a family culture of illness behaviour, she had undergone lengthy treatment in hospital as a young woman and remembered this as the only time her parents had been nice to her. The mother had no medical or nursing training. David's father was assessed to be unsupportive to his wife and uninvolved with the children. The mother's main support appeared to come from her parents-in-law.

In their discussion, one of the areas focused upon by the authors is the role of doctors in the series of events, the story of the mother leading to the FII, harm to the child and the removal of the child from the parental home. They point out (perhaps with surprise) that the problems of anorexia and depression had been treated mainly by sedation. As a young woman, with a poor sense of self-worth and young children, she longed for recognition and affirmation, which her husband was unable to supply. One of the consequences had been difficulties in parenting including experience of the children's behaviour as oppositional. There had been referrals to child psychiatry services with the two older boys. The authors note that this is a common scenario in the clinic: a relatively unsupported mother with low self-esteem struggling to manage her children, unable to access support from her husband and in a stressed marriage.

Unable to have her needs met at home, the mother may have her needs at least partially met by the doctor, in this case with a focus from David's various illnesses. Taking a systemic perspective the 'father's role is to allow this to happen'. He remains outside of the **mother – sick child – doctor** triangle. In addition to this process which meets some needs, presumably subconscious psychological mechanisms influence the illness induction, perhaps as a form of revenge for earlier maltreatment. The object of the revenge could be both the doctor and the child.

In summary a dysfunctional family system becomes replaced, from the child's perspective, by a dysfunctional medical system. The implications for doctors are highlighted including the need in training to bridge the gap between medical and psychological aspects of disease and the value of learning about psychiatric liaison services.

Early life experiences and family patterns of fabricators

A number of authors have reported that fabricating mothers had given a history of abuse in their own childhoods. It is difficult to know what weight should be placed on these histories with regard to their veracity. There could be reporting bias in two directions. Firstly, the actual prevalence of an abuse history could be greater than that reported because of the effect of the nature and strength of psychological defences on the ability to remember, recognize and recount any abuse. Secondly, a perpetrator, upon discovery, may wish to encourage a sympathetic response from professionals and family, and may invent or exaggerate a history of abuse, just as they have invented or exaggerated other things.

Whilst keeping these possible biases in mind, a number of authors have reported a history of sexual abuse (Feldman *et al.*, 1989; Griffith, 1988; McGuire and Feldman, 1989; Wood *et al.*, 1989), physical abuse (Ackerman and Strobel, 1981; Black, 1981; Fialkov, 1984; Geelhoed and Pemberton, 1985; Jones, 1983; Stankler, 1977; Wood *et al.*, 1989) that usually incorporated forms of emotional abuse. In addition Alexander *et al.* (1990) reported that the perpetrator of fabrication had been a victim of rape.

The question of whether a history of neglect or abuse in childhood increases the likelihood of developing a somatizing disorder as an adult and the likelihood of fabricating or inducing illness in a child is a complex issue. The first part of the question was addressed in the south London somatization study referred to in the preceding chapter.

The report by Black (1981) illustrates the effect of a difficult childhood (including physical violence by her father and unsatisfactory relationship with each parent) and the early perceived benefit of 'being ill' which protected her from her father's violence and increased her mother's concern. Thus the childhood experience and the early use of adopting the *sick role* as a child significantly contributed to the development of *somatization* as an adult, including Factitious Disorders in the mother herself, and later FII affecting all three of her children. The paper also indicates the potential for supportive psychotherapy and the possible benefits for the children as a result.

A 30-year-old woman reporting intermittent depression was referred for psychiatric assessment. She complained of anxiety, feelings of irritation and aggression towards her husband and children, and described visual pseudo-hallucinations of her deceased first husband. Although the woman initially gave no psychiatric history, there was a florid medical history of multiple renal, gynaecological and neurological problems. In addition, she claimed to have had abnormal pregnancies and deliveries, and made claims of serious illness for two of her children: agammaglobulinaemia and pyelonephritis.

When the medical notes were studied they revealed that the woman had been under the care of 22 consultants and had been admitted to five hospitals on 30 occasions, of which 10 had been emergencies. The medical histories given by the woman were noted to be distorted and exaggerated at each new referral. The same applied to the family history she had given about both her parents and her children. A psychiatric history was also revealed. There had been two admissions to psychiatric hospital and two brief outpatient episodes. The latter had followed claimed overdoses, although on each occasion there had been no biochemical evidence of ingestion of the substances claimed.

The background included parental marital discord and physical violence by her father to both herself and her mother. The woman expressed dislike of her father and little emotion towards her mother. During childhood she had learnt that 'being ill' protected her from her father's violence and increased her mother's concern for her.

There were two children from the first marriage (her husband died in an accident) and one child from her second marriage. There were substantial difficulties in each marriage. The first husband had been an immature demanding young man. Although the woman described her second husband as more dependable she compared him unfavourably with the first. She perceived him to fail to provide her with overt affection and emotional support. Following the birth of the third child there was a pattern of presenting the children to hospital leading to many emergency admissions to paediatric wards. In the interviews with the psychiatrist the woman expressed no feelings of affection towards her children, but focused on their frequent illnesses and the anxiety this had created.

The intervention consisted of allocating a social worker to the family to provide domiciliary support, placing the children's names on the 'child protection register', and alerting the GP to the situation. The mother participated in supportive psychotherapy with the psychiatrist (author of the paper) at 4–6 week intervals. After one year none of the children or the woman had been admitted to hospital and the children appeared to have escaped further physical harm.

Trans-generational attachment

Whilst the psychiatric disorders identified in perpetrators discussed above are helpful, they provide only a contribution to gaining an understanding of the perpetrator. A number of authors have emphasized that *attention seeking*, and a *strong desire to assume the sick role*, are important motivations, however, as stated by Adshead and Bluglass (2001) the establishing of *motivation* for harmful or deviant behaviour is far from simple and cannot be inferred from behaviour alone. They go on to suggest that in FII the carer's behaviour might be described as '*morbid care giving*', developing an idea illustrated by the phrase '*morbid care eliciting*' used by Henderson in 1974, which he suggested was a process occurring in a variety of psychiatric conditions.

The paper reports how use of a structured interview tool, the adult attachment interview (AAI), was used with both a perpetrating mother and the maternal grandmother. The mother had presented a child with episodes of apnoea (cessation of breathing) and had been inducing these episodes by smothering the child. The mother was rated using the AAI as 'insecure and dismissing' in her pattern of attachment, which was based on her own report of her experience of being parented. Important elements were that she perceived her own mother as having been rejecting and unloving although also there was idealization of her mother. The grandmother presented a more complex picture of attachment, also with a report of her mother as rejecting and unloving. The grandmother presented evidence of an unresolved grief reaction and physical abuse by her father.

The mother had also worked as a professional carer, working in an elderly persons' home, which Adshead and Bluglass (2001) state is consistent with Bowlby's argument (in *Attachment and Loss*, Bowlby, 1969) that insecure attachment may manifest as *'compulsive care giving'*. The history of taking an overdose also fitted with the idea of *'abnormal care-eliciting behaviour'*. In addition, the mother had been perceived by her mother as an ill child and had been presented to doctors on many occasions. For the grandmother also there were indicators of *abnormal care-giving* and *abnormal care-eliciting behaviours*.

The attachment theories put forward by Bowlby are helpful in understanding how the experience of being parented by one generation substantially contributes to how the next generation is parented. The key to the trans-generational (or intergenerational) process is the formation of an 'internal working model' in the mind of the developing child, which is then the basis on which, when the child becomes an adult, she/he parents her/his child. The model has both cognitive and affective components. These components will be linked and the latter may be extremely powerful. With regard to the *internal working model* of the mother, her dismissal of her own lack of care in the attachment narrative (elicited for rating the AAI), and her emphasis on absence of memory as a strategy for dealing with distress, are suggested to indicate how she was able to dismiss the distress of the child.

The authors suggest that limitations of the attachment theories in understanding FII are that it does not address:

- gender role stereotypes and the role of women as caregivers
- the conscious hostility observed in some perpetrators
- the apparent conscious satisfaction of deceiving others
- that disorganized and insecure attachments can be compatible with adequate and non-abusive parenting.

Dimensions of parent behaviour

Eminson and Postlethwaite (1992) present an analysis of FII (MSP) which involves a categorization of parental behaviour in terms of two dimensions:

- a desire to consult
- the ability to distinguish the child's needs from the parents' own needs.

The model is presented in diagrammatic form in Figures 5.2 and 5.3. It can be seen that illness induction is at one extreme of both of these dimensions, i.e. that the desire of the parent to consult is **very high**, and that the ability of the parent to distinguish the needs of the child from their own is **very low** (or non-existent at times) with the result that the parent seeks out healthcare using the extreme method of illness induction. In this situation there would be **little or no agreement** between the parent and the doctor regarding the need for the healthcare.

Eminson and Postlethwaite consider factors that may affect where a parent's behaviour falls on these two dimensions. They point out that there may be a number of factors operating in the following areas:

- in the child
- in the parent
- in the wider family
- in society.

The psychosomatic continuum: what is not FII

There is a spectrum, or continuum, of presentations to medical services of children by their parents when the child is ill, or the child herself or parent believes that the child is ill, or in rare instances when the parent is fabricating or inducing the illness in the child. This continuum between medical illness, *Somatization Disorder* and fabricated (or induced illness) is helpfully discussed and summarized by Krener (1994). When, and to what degree, the child takes on the *sick role* varies amongst individuals, families and cultures. The sick role allows the child, in effect, to take a break from some development tasks (and some regression may occur, especially if the illness is severe or prolonged). This will often be positive and functional allowing the child an opportunity to recover and gradually rejoin their peers in the constant forward movement of the developmental process. Should this movement out of the *sick role* be unduly delayed, or in the unusual situation of FII not actually be necessary, then the child's development is likely to be delayed or even permanently impaired. Consequences may include those listed below in the discussion on the *vulnerable child syndrome*; in particular, an

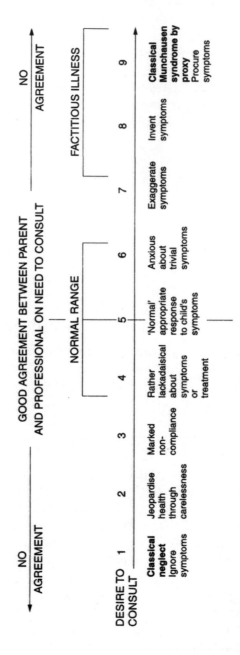

Figure 5.2 Eminson and Postlethwaite's model of 'Parents' desire to consult for their child's symptoms'. Reproduced with permission from *Arch Dis Child* 67: 1510–16; 1992.

9	8	7	6	5
Classical MSP Procured Illness	Invent symptoms	Exaggerate symptoms	Anxious about trivial symptoms	Appropriate concern and response
1	2	3	4	
Classical neglect	Jeopardise health through carelessness	Marked non-compliance	Lackadaisical	

Parents' ability to distinguish child's needs from their own is *seriously compromised* (but may be helped or hindered)

Parents who have *no* ability (at times) to distinguish child's needs from their own

Normal range – parents who *can* and *do* distinguish child's needs from their own

Figure 5.3 The spectrum of healthcare seeking by parents for their child. Table simplified and with notes added, with permission from Eminson and Postlethwaite. *Arch Dis Child* 67: 1510–16; 1992.

8 Frequent presentation for medical attention. Giving medication when virtually no disease and frequently requesting investigations.

7 Insistence on specialist medical attention. Overzealous attention to detail of treatment regimen for existing conditions.

6 Frequent attender at GP for trivial or mild symptoms. Punctilious adherence to treatment and uses medication often.

4 Children have to be quite poorly to be noticed. Lackadaisical re: treatments.

2 Late-presenting ill child. Sporadic attendance and attention to treatments.

aspect of the regression may include a temporary move back to an earlier stage of dependency between the child and the mother, described by Krener and Adelman (1988) as 'a certain fusion of the feelings of the mother and child, a tilt towards non-verbal communication, and special distancing from persons outside the caring dyad'.

There are many contributing factors, both in the child and in the parents, which have an influence on the child moving into and out of the *sick role*. There is a substantial literature on this subject. For the purpose of illuminating the factors that are more relevant to an understanding of FII, this review will focus upon the beliefs and behaviours of the parent in situations when the child is not suffering from any significant organic illness. At this point in the review it is important to state that any movement into or out of the *sick role* almost always involves a two-directional interaction between the patient (and, in the case of the child, the parent as carer) and members of medical services, usually doctors.

Children as well as adults may present with physical symptoms which result from the *somatization* of anxiety and are associated with avoidance of a situation, perhaps most commonly attending school. A successful intervention will include helping the child to deal with their anxiety using psychosocial means (sometimes combined with a medicine). It is almost always necessary to work with the parents of the child. They are likely to benefit from an explanation of the origins of symptoms, advice about how to manage the child and sometimes to work on relationships within the family using formal family therapy. Difficulties may arise if the child avoids the treatment and also if the parents remain unconvinced of the psychological origin of the physical symptoms; this is **not**, however, FII.

The concept of *vulnerability* in a child is set out in a way which is helpful for medical clinicians by Boyce (1992). *Vulnerability* is defined as 'a condition of unusual or exaggerated susceptibility to the environmental agents of disease or disorder, including psychosocial stressors'. He considers the view of the vulnerability of the child according to the physician and compares this with the view of the parent. From this position Boyce presents a two-dimensional model, or taxonomy, which is shown in diagrammatic form in his paper, which is adapted and reproduced here as Figure 5.4.

TRUE VULNERABILITY		
HIGH	LOW	
A chronic disease illness prone child	B vulnerable child syndrome FII	HIGH PARENTAL PERCEPTION OF VULNERABILITY
C child neglect	D normal child	LOW

Figure 5.4   Childhood vulnerability adapted from Boyce (1992). The model is a consideration of the perception of vulnerability of the child compared with the true vulnerability as defined by the paediatrician based on objective information.

It is critically important to emphasize that what is being addressed here is *the idea that the child is vulnerable* in the **mind of the parent**. Accompanying the idea held by the parent will be powerful emotions, although the latter are unlikely to be easily detectable. As the model allows, the child may, or may not, actually be vulnerable in the opinion of an independent assessor, usually a paediatrician. Some of the factors in the child's history may influence the parent's perception of the vulnerability of the child, and this will be associated with the vulnerability of the parent. Thus the more extreme the vulnerability of the parent, including the need to somatize, and the need to receive care by whatever means, including by deception, the more likely it is that FII could develop.

The vulnerable child

The concept of the *vulnerable child* had been introduced into the literature by Green and Solnit in 1964. The hypothesis that 'children who are expected by their parents to die prematurely often react with a disturbance in psycho-social development' is addressed and supported in their paper.

The expectation to die includes three situations:

- children who suffered a serious illness and the parents did not believe that they would recover
- children who represent for the parent, usually the mother, a figure from the past who died prematurely
- children who are expected to die because in their birth the mother's fear of her own dying became displaced on to the baby.

The presenting features of this 'vulnerable child syndrome' are considered in four areas:

- difficulty with separation
- *infantilization*
- bodily over-concerns
- school under-achievement.

Pathological separation difficulties include night-time problems – the parent sleeping close to the child and waking through the night to seek reassurance that the child is still alive. What the authors refer to as *infantilization* involves the parent becoming overprotective, overly indulgent and oversolicitous, while the child is overly dependent, disobedient, irritable, argumentative and uncooperative. Feeding problems are a common accompaniment. There may be bodily over-concerns with child complaining of headaches or abdominal pain, and mother overly concerned about minor symptoms. Older children frequently complain of abdominal pain before school and a classical *school phobia* may be present. School under-achievement may result.

Twelve possible predisposing factors are suggested for a 'vulnerable child syndrome':

1 The child is the first born after the parents have become resigned to childlessness.
2 Congenital abnormality in the child.
3 Premature birth.
4 Acquired disability.
5 The child already has had a truly life-threatening illness.
6 During pregnancy the doctor had predicted that the foetus might die.

7 The mother suffered postpartum depression.
8 The parents are unable to have further children.
9 A previous unresolved grief reaction is present in one of the parents.
10 A hereditary disorder is present in the family.
11 The mother has conscious strongly ambivalent feelings towards the child.
12 There is a psychologic(al) need in the mother to find something physically wrong with the child, a displacement of unacceptable feelings towards the child, or of unacceptable thoughts and reactions associated with the birth of the child.

The authors add that in the latter situation:

> *such a parent repeatedly brings her child for medical attention, usually to many doctors, for a host of complaints because of her* **certainty** *that the child has leukaemia, a brain tumour, or some other elusive malignant disease, even though a succession of doctors have been unable to make a diagnosis.*

This paper, and the concept of the *vulnerable child*, are of interest, not only because of the discussion about unusual beliefs about the state of health of the child, but also about associated over-protection and separation difficulties. All of these features may occur also when illness is being fabricated.

Illness behaviour and abnormal illness behaviour

Illness behaviour concerns how people think and behave when they are, or think they are, or might be, ill. Mechanic (1962), a sociologist, approached the subject of illness behaviour from the perspective of public health and medical sociology, and much of his life's work has concerned aspects of healthcare systems. One objective was to understand 'the influence of a variety of norms, values, fears, and expected rewards and punishments on how a symptomatic person behaves'. The concept of **illness behaviour** was proposed, by which Mechanic referred to 'the ways in which given symptoms may be differentially perceived, evaluated and acted upon (or not acted upon) by different kinds of persons'.

Pilowsky, a psychiatrist taking a clinical perspective, has written a series of papers on the evolving subject of what he termed abnormal illness behaviour. Initially (1969) he reviewed this concept from the starting position of the physician who faces a patient with physical complaints for which no adequate organic cause can be found. A range of possible (psychiatric) diagnostic labels may be applied in such a situation. Pilowsky (1989) defined abnormal illness behaviour as:

> *the persistence of an inappropriate or maladaptive mode of perceiving, evaluating, or acting in relation to one's own state of health, despite the fact that a doctor (or other appropriate social agent) has offered an accurate and reasonably lucid explanation of the nature of the illness and the appropriate course of management to be followed (if any), with opportunities for discussion, negotiation and clarification based on adequate assessment of all biological, psychological, social and cultural factors.*

The importance of the explanation offered by the doctor raises the questions of accuracy and lucidity in the context of a matching between the understanding of the doctor and of the patient. For example, problems may arise if there are significant differences in the use of language, intellect, ethnicity and culture, especially if these differences are poorly appreciated by the doctor.

What is somatization?

According to Kleinman and Kleinman (1985) somatization is 'the expression of personal and social distress in an idiom of bodily complaints with medical help seeking'. Lipowski (1988) wrote that somatization 'is the tendency to experience and communicate somatic distress in response to psychosocial stress and to seek medical help for it'. And with regard to the implications he stated that somatization 'poses a major, medical, social, and economic problem'.

What is Somatization Disorder?

Somatization Disorder (SD) is a psychiatric diagnosis in both of the major systems of classification of mental disorders: the ICD in Europe and the DSM in the USA. The systems are very similar although a few minor differences exist in terminology and the scheme of classification, so the Appendix provides a list of disorders according to both systems. Essentially the diagnosis of SD is made when there have been multiple, recurrent, and frequently changing physical symptoms over several years. The diagnosis has been widely adopted in the USA with lifetime prevalence rates ranging from 0.2% to 2% among women and less than 0.2% in men (American Psychiatric Association, 1994).

A number of authoritative workers have put forward the view that, for clinical purposes, the diagnostic criteria for **SD** are rather restrictive because in the context of a number of studies the incidence of patients meeting some of the criteria and having high consultation rates was found to be many times that of those meeting the strict criteria for SD. Gill and Bass (1997) suggested that *Undifferentiated Somatization Disorder* (a form with less strict diagnostic criteria) is about 100 times more common than **SD**, noting that these constitute about 20% of new consultations in primary care.

What influences the development of somatization?

The south London somatization study looked at the incidence of **somatization** in an urban population (Craig *et al.*, 1993 and 1994). One of the findings concerned evidence regarding the origins of somatizing disorders. The researchers suggested that lack of parental care, followed by childhood illness, contribute to two separate pathways, which come together in childhood and lead to **somatization** in adulthood. Using this model the lack of parental care would increase the risk that the individual would suffer from an emotional disorder (in response to certain stressful situations) and the early exposure to illness would predispose the individual to interpret the bodily sensations as symptoms of serious illness. The combination is the critical feature, since neither of these antecedents alone accounted for the **somatization** in adulthood. The results also suggest that *acute* somatization is best viewed as a particularly common manifestation of emotional disorder in general practice. Individuals who went on to present with chronic somatization more often initially presented with symptoms that had no psycho-physiological basis (for example, no symptoms of anxiety such as palpitations).

References

Ackerman NB, Strobel CT. Polle syndrome: chronic diarrhea in Munchausen's child. *Gastroenterology*. 1981; 81(6): 1140–2.

Adshead G, Bluglass K. A vicious circle: transgenerational attachment representations in a case of factitious illness by proxy. *Attachment and Human Development*. 2001; 3(1): 77–95.

Alexander R, Smith W, Stevenson R. Serial Munchausen syndrome by proxy. *Pediatrics*. 1990; 86(4): 581–5.

American Psychiatric Association. *Diagnostic and Statistical Manual of Mental Disorder (Fourth Edition) DSM-IV*. Washington DC: American Psychiatric Association; 1994.

Black D. The extended Munchausen syndrome: a family case. *British Journal of Psychiatry*. 1981; 138: 466–9.

Bowlby J. *Attachment and Loss. Vol. 1 Attachment*. London: Hogarth Press and the Institute of Psychoanalysis; 1969.

Boyce WT. The vulnerable child: new evidence, new approaches. *Advanced Paediatrics*. 1992; 39: 1–33.

Craig TK, Boardman AP, Mills K, Daly-Jones O, Drake H. The south London somatization study. I: Longitudinal course and the influence of early life experience. *British J Psychiatry*. 1993; 163: 579–88.

Craig TK, Drake H, Mills K, Boardman AP. The south London somatization study. II: Influence of stressful life events, and secondary gain. *British J Psychiatry*. 1994; 165: 248–58.

Eminson DM, Postlethwaite RJ. Factitious illness: recognition and management. *Archives of Disease in Childhood*. 1992; 67: 1510–16.

Feldman KW, Christopher DM, Opheim KB. Munchausen syndrome/bulimia by proxy: ipecac as a toxin in child abuse. *Child Abuse and Neglect*. 1989; 13: 257–61.

Fialkov MJ. Peregrination in the problem pediatric patient: the pediatric Munchhausen syndrome? *Clinical Pediatrics*. 1984; 23(10): 571–5.

Geelhoed GC, Pemberton PJ. SIDS, seizures or 'sophageal reflux? Another manifestation of Munchausen syndrome by proxy. *Medical Journal of Australia*. 1985; 143(8): 357–8.

Gill D, Bass C. Somatoform and dissociative disorders: assessment and treatment. *Advances in Psychiatric Treatment*. 1997; 3: 9–16.

Gray J, Bentovim A. Illness induction syndrome: paper I – a series of 41 children from 37 families identified at the Great Ormond Street Hospital for Children NHS Trust. *Child Abuse and Neglect*. 1996; 20: 655–73.

Green M, Solnit AJ. Reactions to the loss of a child: a vulnerable child syndrome. *Pediatrics*. 1964; 34: 58–66.

Griffith JL. The family systems of Munchausen syndrome by proxy. *Family Process*. 1988; 27: 423–37.

Henderson S. Care-eliciting behaviour in man. *J Nervous and Mental Disease*. 1974; 159: 172–81.

Jones DPH. Dermatitis artefacta in mother and baby as child abuse. *British Journal of Psychiatry*. 1983; 143: 199–200.

Kleinman A, Kleinman J. Somatisation: the interconnections in Chinese society among culture, depressive experiences, and the meanings of pain. In: Kleinman A, Good B, editors. *Culture and Depression*. Berkeley, CA: University of California; 1985.

Krener P. Factitious disorders and the psychosomatic continuum in children. *Current Opinion in Pediatrics*. 1994; **6**: 418–22.

Krener P, Adelman R. Parent salvage and parent sabotage in the care of chronically ill children. *American Journal of Diseases of Children*. 1988; **142**(9): 945–51.

Lipowski ZJ. Somatization: the concept and its clinical application. *American Journal of Psychiatry*. 1988; **145**(11): 1358–68.

Loader P, Kelly C. Munchausen Syndrome by Proxy: a narrative approach to explanation. *Clinical Child Psychology and Psychiatry*. 1996; **1**: 353–63.

McGuire TL, Feldman KW. Psychologic morbidity of children subjected to Munchausen syndrome by proxy. *Pediatrics*. 1989; **83**(2): 289–92.

Mechanic D. The concept of illness behaviour. *J Chronic Disease*. 1962; **15**: 189–94.

Pilowsky I. Abnormal illness behaviour. *British Journal of Medical Psychology*. 1969; **42**: 347–51.

Pilowsky I. Illness behaviour and neuroses. *Current Opinion in Psychiatry*. 1989; **2**: 217–24.

Stankler L. Factitious skin lesions in a mother and two sons. *British Journal of Dermatology*. 1977; **97**: 217–19.

Wood PR, Fowlkes J, Holden P, Casto D. Fever of unknown origin for six years: Munchausen syndrome by proxy (clinical conference). *Journal of Family Practice*. 1989; **28**: 391–5.

Further reading

Hardwick P. Health beliefs and myths in child and adolescent practice. *Clinical Child Psychology Psychiatry*. 1998; **3**: 87–102.

Hardwick PJ. Families' medical myths. *Journal of Family Therapy*. 1989; **11**: 3–27.

Mechanic D. The influence of mothers on their children's health attitudes and behavior. *Pediatrics*. 1964; **33**: 444–53.

Mechanic D. The concept of illness behaviour: culture, situation and personal predisposition. *Psychological Medicine*. 1986; **16**: 1–7.

Parsons T. *The Social System*. New York: The Free Press; 1951.

Chapter 6

Responses by professionals: challenges for the multi-disciplinary response

Section headings
Policy and practice
The starting position
Uncertainty in FII
Degree of certainty of the diagnosis of fabrication or induction
Addressing particular difficulties in managing FII
Developing good inter-agency practice
Implications for training
KEY WORDS
Children Act 1989
Physical harm
Psychological harm
Persuasive denial
Polarization in case management
Multi-disciplinary response

Policy and practice

The Government Guidance *Safeguarding Children in Whom Illness is Fabricated or Induced* (HM Government, 2007) sets out principles and processes for agencies and professionals to manage a suspected case of FII. This is addressed within the framework of the Children Act 1989 and other Government Guidance concerning the management of child abuse. Even with the help of such comprehensive guidance, management of FII often remains difficult and a number of particular challenges and dilemmas face professionals. For some the challenge will be a once-in-a-lifetime experience, and for others, perhaps working in a specialist paediatric setting, various presentations of FII may provide recurring challenges. The purpose of this chapter is to draw attention to some of the particular difficulties that may be encountered by professionals when dealing with FII and present some ways forward that have been suggested by professionals. The importance of inter-agency and multi-disciplinary working is emphasized, which is critical to achieve the best outcome for the child in whom illness has been induced or fabricated.

The starting position

Management needs to address the issues that are specific to FII. Issues concerning the child, and the behaviour and psychopathology of the fabricator, have been addressed in the early chapters of this publication and it is important to be well informed about these and to understand their implications for management. What follows is a distillation with key points concerning the child and the fabricator.

Key issues concerning the child

- In the short term the child may be at risk of suffering from physical harm. The situation may progress to more serious levels of harm, including the risk of death.
- Harm to the child may have already occurred in the time before the identification of the fabrication (*see* the evidence from co-morbidity studies; failure to thrive, inappropriate medication, impaired psychological development) although it may be difficult to clarify with certainty.
- In the medium term the risks of harm, or even death, are likely to continue without a decisive intervention.
- In the long term there is the likelihood of impairment of the child's overall development: even without physical harm, the risk of psychological harm is significant.
- A young victim may be unable to verbalize or indicate what is happening.
- An older child may have become 'numbed' by the continuing experience of 'living a lie of illness' and appear, at least superficially, to be collusive with the fabricator.

Key issues concerning the fabricator

- The fabricator may appear to have a close and caring relationship with the child; the relationship with the child may actually be cold and uncaring.
- The fabricator may be friendly with professional staff even to the extent of building personal relationships.
- A setting for the FII may be a history of lying and deception of various sorts.

- The fabricator is likely to have a history of Somatizing Disorder, but this is not necessarily the case.
- The behaviours of the fabricator may be strongly driven by a belief system that the child **must have** something physically wrong.
- The fabricator may, in a state of desperation, escalate the fabricating behaviours or discharge the child from hospital (in the latter case only to later seek a further opinion elsewhere).
- The fabricator may use excessively particular psychological mechanisms, which are at risk of adversely affecting the professionals (these are addressed specifically below).

Uncertainty in FII

In perhaps all presentations of FII there will be a number of areas of uncertainty to be considered. The central, or overarching, uncertainties are likely to be:

- whether harm has been/is occurring as a result of parental action
- the risk of future harm
- boundaries between abuse and other medical and treatment dilemmas.

There are two phases of uncertainty which relate to the process of decision-making. Initially uncertainties will arise as part of the process of deciding if it is indeed FII that is being encountered. Then it is likely that there will be uncertainties about the most appropriate next step in management. Issues contributing to these areas of uncertainty as discussed in 'Dealing with uncertainty' (Baildam and Eminson, 2000) are summarized in Table 6.1, tabulated and divided into the two phases.

The authors of the above suggest four ways in which to deal with situations of uncertainty.

1 Clarify which specific areas of harm are to be further considered – keep in mind short or longer term, physical and psychological risks.
2 Take the issue outside of the simple doctor–patient relationship – share concerns with others (e.g. colleague, a professional with

Table 6.1 Issues contributing to uncertainty in FII. Summarized from '*Dealing with uncertainty*' by Eileen Baildam and Mary Eminson (2000).

Table 6.1a Possible uncertainties in deciding if FII is present.

Area of uncertainty	Issues, questions and suggestions
Is this fabrication, or something else?	A spectrum exists of parenting behaviour in relation to child health and illness. Illness induction is at the extreme of a spectrum of behaviours. Verbal fabrication may be more difficult to recognize.
Unfamiliar areas of history taking may be required to ascertain facts.	Multiple sources of information may be needed. It may help to link parent and child (and possibly sibling) histories.
FII is likely to involve lack of normal trust between parent and doctor. If the child is disabled.	The doctor will need to deal with uncomfortable emotions. Uncertainty regarding symptoms and signs in the presence of multiple physical problems which constitute the disability, or if learning disability is present.
If the child is older or adolescent.	Has there been coaching or collusion? Does the child now have his/her own Somatization Disorder?
Cultural issues.	Norms are culture bound. There is variation of response to illness, or threat of illness, in different cultures.

Table 6.1b Possible uncertainties in deciding appropriate management.

Area of uncertainty	Issues, questions and suggestions
Lack of clarity by professionals about responsibility to the child.	Primacy of the rights and needs of the child. Tension with the rights and needs of the parent.
If the parent has mental health problems.	Uncertainty about appropriate use of legal action to protect the child. Childcare legislation or Mental Health Act?
Lack of uniformity in judgement of risk and subsequent management amongst professionals.	Considerable variation has been noted in opinions concerning the ongoing risk to children by professional teams and Local Authorities.
Non-consent to psychiatric involvement by the family.	Removes a potential way forward to assist the child and family. Is it a reasonable position?

more specialist knowledge, a medico-legal expert, an 'emotional abuse panel', a hospital ethics committee).
3 Widen the knowledge base – by gathering more contextual information perhaps from primary care professionals.
4 Reappraisal of the literature – appreciate the heterogeneous nature of subjects in studies of outcome.

Degree of certainty of the diagnosis of fabrication or induction

Rosenberg (2003) takes a pragmatic and clear approach to the 'degree of certainty' of a *medical diagnosis* of fabrication or induction. In a discussion about the process of diagnosis by inclusion and by exclusion of certain features she presents four main categories of the degree of certainty of the diagnosis:

1a definitive diagnosis by inclusion
1b definitive diagnosis by exclusion
2 possible diagnosis
3 inconclusive determination
4 definitely not fabrication – the diagnosis is excluded by another explanation.

It is emphasized that the criteria refer to medical (paediatric) diagnosis and that the intent, or the psychiatric status, of the perpetrator is of no relevance to this process. Rosenberg adds however that 'this does not diminish the importance, indeed the centrality, of mental health professionals' when the diagnosis is under consideration, and the necessity for paediatric and mental health professionals to work closely together. The reasons for involvement of the mental health professionals may relate to the needs of the fabricator, the victim and the network of professionals.

Addressing particular difficulties in managing FII

Two papers usefully address the problems.

Waller (1983) addresses the issues that arise from the often-found features of FII. Waller emphasizes the link, and similarity with, what had been reported on and termed 'non-accidental poisoning' (or 'the chemically abused child' by Shnaps *et al.*, in 1981). He also highlights obstacles to treatment and how a consulting psychiatrist may be able to assist in dealing with these.

The case reported included a fabricated history of easy bruising, vomiting, and coughing up blood. The samples of blood provided by the mother, supposedly from the child, were proven to originate from the mother. The first obstacle to treatment had been overcome by an alert and informed haematologist. The second obstacle is appreciating that verbal fabrication can progress to illness induction, as in non-accidental poisoning: a progression from apparent disease to actual disease. A key point from the paper included the follow-up of a child, previously reported by other authors (Kurlandsky *et al.*, 1979), who remained with the perpetrating parent, and at follow-up had died (information obtained from a personal communication with Kessler, 1980). The initial fabrications were of bleeding and later there was actual apnoea presumably due to airway obstruction due to introduced blood.

Waller reviews 23 earlier published reports of non-accidental poisoning and points out that at least five of the 23 children were known to have died. The prominent themes identified included:

> *recurrent illnesses in the mothers, or involvement in some aspect of the medical or nursing profession; valid reasons based on past events for the mothers to be especially concerned for their children's health; and evidence of profound depression which becomes apparent only after their behaviour in making the child appear ill has been blocked.*

The third obstacle was described as the 'rather startling tie' between the parent and the child. Waller was struck by the presence of separation anxiety and over-protectiveness in the case he describes. The child as well as the mother displayed these features and for this reason Waller refers to 'the symbiotic bond' between mother and child. The use of the term 'symbiotic bond' to refer to the relationship between the parent and child is an interesting one. In FII it is the children who in some way help their parent to deal with their own psychological and medical concerns. This author prefers not to use the term symbiotic, which biologists use to refer to a relationship which is mutually beneficial to each contributor, as in FII it is difficult to see the benefits for the child.

The fourth obstacle is the highly persuasive denial on the part of the parents when confronted with the situation. Waller states that:

> the disturbance in thought content and behaviour may be a dissociative phenomenon, or a form of pseudologia fantastica (pathological lying), in which the parent comes to believe, at least intermittently, the fantasy that the child has a primary, rather than a fabricated illness.

The fifth obstacle reported by Waller was the disbelief in the legal system and the understandable scepticism on the part of legal authorities when asked to intervene on behalf of the child. This problem was perhaps more evident at the time of publication (1983 in Texas, USA) than at present.

Freeland and Foley (1992) from Australia address the achievement of effective case management of FII by a social work team. They consider the problem of potential polarization between the desire to engage the family and to confront the denial. These two processes may be seen as mutually exclusive. Applying systemic thinking they form eight propositions, which are listed below.

- Because of the potential danger of serious physical abuse to the children, the level of responsibility taken by the professionals for protection of the child should be inversely related to the level of responsibility taken by the parents.
- When attempting to establish the existence of the syndrome (i.e. FII), the vigour with which assessment information is sought needs to be greater than the apparent resistance of the parents to disclose.
- Workers tend to deal with dependency in polarized ways.
- Non-intrusive protective options become less viable with more serious abuse and more entrenched behaviour patterns in the perpetrator.
- The complexity of the system constructed by the workers, for effective intervention, mirrors the complexity of the abuse.
- The level of teamwork and cooperation is proportional to the permeability of the boundaries between different professional disciplines and within levels of bureaucracy.

- The degree of cohesion and commitment of the team members is also related to the level of disclosure of information and self-disclosure of doubts, issues and problems experienced by team members.
- In the final analysis, the commitment of the workers to teamwork and multi-disciplinary intervention needs to be greater than the abusing parent's compulsion to abuse and avoid detection of that abuse.

Developing good inter-agency practice

Horwath (1999) considers the difficulties in the management, which occur at personal, professional and organizational levels, as a result of tensions and dilemmas which are especially prominent when managing cases of FII.

Horwath focuses on inter-agency working and concludes from an overview of the literature that 'the lack of distinctive features and lack of consensus regarding case management create a number of dilemmas for professionals. This in turn inhibits effective inter-agency practice'.

The five dilemmas or areas of debate centre around the following issues:

1 Is the child sick or abused? At what stage do medical personnel acknowledge that they may not be dealing with a sick child but with a possible case of child abuse?
2 Should all professionals work together as equals or should one professional or group of professionals take lead responsibility for the FII assessment?
3 How can one protect a child and work in partnership with a suspected perpetrator of FII and their family?
4 Can professionals working with a suspected case of FII balance the rights of the child with the rights of the parent?
5 Does the perpetrator require care or control? Is the mother suffering from a mental illness or is she an instigator of a criminal act?

Horwath concluded that the ACPC child protection procedures in place at the time of writing in 1999, were unlikely to provide the framework required for effective professional practice when attempting to address the unique problems presented by cases of FII. Horwath stated that this may be achieved by developing policies, guidelines and procedures that enable managers and practitioners to define aims and objectives, identify methods of intervention, and clarify roles and responsibilities. These statements were made, however, before the publication of the Government Guidance, *Safeguarding Children in Whom Illness is Fabricated or Induced* (DH *et al.*, 2002).

Specific recommendations were that guidance was required on the following:

- procedures for exploring concerns, sharing information and initiating informal discussions between professionals; these should recognize that in the early stages of investigating these cases it may not always be appropriate to begin a formal child protection investigation
- key professionals with whom concerns should be shared
- the management of the initial child protection conference; for example, which, if any, family members should be invited?
- appointment of a case coordinator who would act as a focal point for gathering and collating information and coordinating interventions
- protocols for recording information
- the use of covert video surveillance
- working in 'partnership' with the alleged perpetrator and family members
- complaints procedures.

These issues are addressed in the Guidance issued by the Government in 2002 and reissued in 2007. The accompanying training pack will facilitate their use in practice.

Parrish and Perman (2004) from the USA also address the need for a carefully organized inter-disciplinary response. They draw attention to the importance of the role of the social worker and that this has been historically under-considered in the existing literature. Helpfully and critically the authors keep the focus on the child in the face of what is likely to be a potentially unclear situation. The primary goal of both short-term and long-term treatment must be to first address the protection of the child from further harm. Box 6.1 is particularly helpful as an *aide mémoire* of considerations, including attachment, kinship, and long-term issues and is reproduced here in a slightly modified form.

Box 6.1   Clinical considerations regarding children following identification of FII

- The child's developmental stage and level of attachment.
- Availability of suitable, safe kinship care.
- Availability of therapeutic foster care.
- Risks of additional trauma caused by separation from siblings and other familiar individuals.
- Long-term implications for attachment.
- Long-term implications for child's mental health profile, including risks of Factitious Disorder.
- Questions of inter-generational replication of FII.

(From Parish and Perman, 2004.)

Implications for training

A practically helpful review article by Horwath (2003) takes an overview of the development of good practice and **implications for training**.

Whilst the three government guidance documents (*Working Together to Safeguard Children*, HM Government, 2006; *Framework for the Assessment of Children in Need and their Families*, DH *et al.*, 2000; and *Safeguarding Children in Whom Illness is Fabricated or Induced*, HM Government, 2007) are essential, useful and welcome it is important to recognize that 'processes and procedures are never ends in themselves, but should always be used as a means of bringing about better outcomes for children' (HM Government, 2007). Inter-agency training is one cornerstone of developing good practice.

Essentially three levels of training are identified for:

- those in contact with children
- those who work directly with children, or with adults who are parents

- those involved in assessment and intervention to safeguard children.

At the basic level all must be aware of the ways in which FII may present and how to ensure safe practice. From level two a practical knowledge is required of *Working Together to Safeguard Children*, and *Safeguarding Children in Whom Illness is Fabricated or Induced*. At the third level professionals should understand fully the *Assessment Framework* and some training in court skills is required. A key issue is attitudinal shift among professionals, who need to recognize **the importance of interdependence.** Inter-agency training can go some way towards promoting collaborative practice and interdependence. However, there may be particular issues for professionals who traditionally work alone, for example medical GPs, and in such cases a flexible approach to training tailored to the needs of the individual may be required.

For professionals identifying and working with FII (including paediatricians, police in child protection units and social workers) suggested areas to be covered were:

- presentation of FII including physical and emotional presentations
- epidemiology, current research and outcomes
- personal and professional responses to FII and their potential impact on practice
- specialist professional roles (for example, the use of covert video surveillance for police officers)
- the role of the organization and available resources
- issues of confidentiality and working together with the child and family.

These areas will be covered in either or both of this Reader and the accompanying training pack.

Finally Horwath (2003) addresses the possible personal and professional responses to FII that may potentially affect practice. Horwath draws attention to the survey carried out by the Royal College of Paediatrics and Child Health. The College reported that the sense of anxiety generated by FII could lead to one of three broad types of response:

- running away, denying that the child may be a victim of FII

- holding extreme viewpoints – for example, that certain paediatricians are 'on an FII bandwagon' and over-diagnose
- attempting to find realistic ways of managing cases of FII.

There is no reason to think that these types of response will not
also be present in other professionals who encounter FII. Horwath
states that the needs of professionals who respond in the first two
ways are unlikely to be met through training and suggests that
these types of anxiety should be managed through supervision
(Horwath refers to Morrison, 2001).

References

Baildam E, Eminson M. Dealing with uncertainty. In: Eminson M,
Postlethwaite RJ, editors. *Munchausen Syndrome by Proxy Abuse: a practical
approach*. Oxford: Butterworth Heinemann; 2000. Out of print but pdf
available on *Incredibly Caring*. Oxford: Radcliffe Publishing; 2007.

Department of Health, Home Office, Department for Education and Skills,
Welsh Assembly Government. *Safeguarding Children in Whom Illness is Fabricated or Induced*. London: Department of Health Publications; 2002.
www.doh.gov.uk/qualityprotects

Department of Health, Department for Education and Employment and the
Home Office. *Framework for the Assessment of Children in Need and their
Families*. London: The Stationery Office; 2000.

Freeland H, Foley S. The management of polarisation in Munchausen syndrome by proxy. In: Calvert G, Ford A, Parkinson P, editors. *The Practice of
Child Protection: Australian approaches*. Sydney: Hale and Iremonger; 1992.

HM Government. *Working Together to Safeguard Children: a guide for interagency
working to safeguard and promote the welfare of children*. London: The Stationery
Office; 2006.

HM Government. *Safeguarding Children in Whom Illness is Fabricated or Induced*.
London: Department for Education and Skills; 2007. www.everychildmatters.
gov.uk/safeguarding

Horwath J. Inter-agency practice in suspected cases of Munchausen syndrome
by proxy (Fictitious illness by proxy): dilemmas for professionals. *Child and
Family Social Work*. 1999; **4**: 109–18.

Horwath J. Developing good practice in cases of fabricated and induced illness
by carers: new guidance and training implications. *Child Abuse Review*. 2003;
12: 58–63.

Kessler RW. Personal communication (1980). Quoted by Waller (1983).

Kurlandsky I, Lukoff JY, Zinkham WH, Brody JP, Kessler RW. Munchausen
syndrome by proxy: definition of factitious bleeding by 51Cr labeling of
erythrocytes. *Pediatrics*. 1979; **63**(2): 228–31.

Morrison T. *Staff Supervision in Social Care. Making a real difference for staff and
service users*. Brighton: Pavilion; 2001.

Parrish M, Perman J. Munchausen syndrome by proxy: some practice implications for social workers. *Child and Adolescent Social Work Journal.* 2004; **21**: 137–54.

Rosenberg D. Munchausen Syndrome by Proxy: medical diagnostic criteria. *Child Abuse and Neglect.* 2003; **27**(4): 421–30.

Shnaps Y, Frand M, Rotem Y, Tirosh M. The chemically abused child. *Pediatrics.* 1981; **61**(1): 119–21.

Waller DA. Obstacles to the treatment of Munchausen by proxy syndrome. *Journal American Academy of Child and Adolescent Psychiatry.* 1983; **22**(1): 80–5.

Further reading

Gray J. The social work role in Munchausen syndrome by proxy. In: Adshead G, Brooke D, editors. *Munchausen's Syndrome by Proxy. Current issues in assessment, treatment and research.* London: Imperial College Press; 2001.

Neale B, Bools C, Meadow R. Problems in the assessment and management of Munchausen syndrome by proxy abuse. *Children and Society.* 1991; **5**: 324–33.

Pearce D, Bools C. The child protection process. In: Eminson M, Postlethwaite RJ, editors. *Munchausen Syndrome by Proxy Abuse: a practical approach.* Oxford: Butterworth Heinemann; 2000. Out of print but pdf available on *Incredibly Caring.* Oxford: Radcliffe Publishing; 2007.

Pizzey S. The role of the guardian ad litem. In: Adshead G, Brooke D, editors. *Munchausen's Syndrome by Proxy. Current issues in assessment, treatment and research.* London: Imperial College Press; 2001.

Sanders MJ. Hospital Protocol for the evaluation of Munchausen syndrome by proxy. *Clinical Child Psychology and Psychiatry.* 1995; **4**: 379–91.

Whelan-Williams S, Baker T. A multidisciplinary hospital response protocol. In: Parnell TF, Day DO. *Munchausen Syndrome by Proxy: misunderstood child abuse.* Thousand Oaks: Sage; 1998.

Chapter 7

Contributions by psychiatric services

Section headings
Overview
Individual psychotherapy as an outpatient
Individual psychotherapy as an inpatient
Family therapy
Outcome of psychiatric intervention
KEY WORDS
Individual psychotherapy
Family therapy

Overview

Whilst acknowledging the difficulties in achieving sufficient engagement to produce a successful outcome (for both child and parent), psychotherapeutic treatment of fabricators is sometimes possible. Given the risks to the child victim of FII described in earlier chapters, the setting for the opportunity for the fabricator to undergo psychiatric treatment will almost always be within a child safeguarding framework. The treatment will be one component of a carefully managed plan delivered by children's social care, psychiatric and other services working together. This chapter aims to present to the reader the possibility of psychiatric treatment by describing examples of successful treatment. The contribution of adult mental health services as well as child and adolescent mental health services (CAMHS) will be considered. We are aware of four papers describing treatment in some detail. In Chapter 5 we have already described treatment using a narrative approach. In this chapter we present two papers describing individual treatments and one describing family treatment. A further successful treatment of a family is briefly mentioned. All were successful. In the first description of individual treatment it is notable that the husband of the fabricator, and father of the child victim, also made significant positive changes even though he was not included in the treatment sessions.

It is perhaps important to emphasize the conditions under which these successful treatments occurred which were common to the different settings and methods of therapy. In all cases there was:

- acknowledgement (perhaps not initially, but by degree and in time) of the fabrication and behaviour harmful to the child
- commitment by the perpetrator to therapeutic work leading to change
- sufficient professional resources to offer long-term monitoring and support as well as the initial phase of intensive therapy.

Individual psychotherapy as an outpatient

The earliest report of individual psychotherapeutic treatment was by Nicol and Eccles (1985). Two children from a family of four children were presented with FII. The youngest, the only girl, had been subjected to life-threatening illness induction by salt poisoning from the age of 10 weeks. Subsequently over the following 12 months the child had been admitted to hospital on another 11 occasions. This amounted to 29 weeks in hospital, which was 43% of her life at that time.

An important point was that the mother acknowledged the illness induction after being informed that the decision of a Child Protection Case Conference was to remove the child to foster care: at that point the professionals were hopeful about the possibility of treatment for the mother. Following attendance at court and the making of a Care Order, the child was returned home under 'very strict social work and health visitor supervision' and a trial of psychotherapy was undertaken.

The mother had a history of frequent attendance at the GP. After a few sessions of therapy by a child psychiatrist it became clear that the mother had a strong wish to understand herself, she was intelligent and had a capacity to bring active and painful feelings to therapy sessions. The initial decision to commence with supportive therapy was modified, and a more active and deeper form of interpretive therapy was undertaken. Therapy thus continued for six months with weekly sessions and then for a further six months fortnightly. Although the individual therapy was ended, family supervision by the social worker and health visitor continued.

Nicol and Eccles distilled out the main themes of the therapy and summarized these as follows.

Presentation – the mother attended on time and was always well presented. The mother indicated that she had continued to think about issues in the intervals between the sessions.

The reason for the abuse – complex motives emerged including liking the sympathy and feeling of importance when the child was on the hospital ward. She liked contact with the doctors although at the same time enjoyed the feeling that she had outwitted them. Full realization of the danger she had put her child in emerged.

Affective expression in therapy – two important affective states emerged; remorse and something the patient called 'depression'. At one stage the former led to lying awake at night contemplating what she had done. The depression was not considered to be clinical depression: it was an unpleasant mood-state that later seemed to have infantile rage as a central component, together with crushingly low self-esteem.

The pathway to the abuse – although the deception was totally conscious there was a deeper disturbance responsible for the motivations. The woman's parents were quite extreme in their roles within the family. Her father had been a bully and her mother timid and placating with a chronic over-concern about her own and her children's health. The woman failed academically and went to work in the local town hall, where she met her future husband. The woman's idealization of her father was tested when he had been drinking heavily, was sacked from work and eventually appeared in court for dangerous driving. The woman reported feeling depressed for the first time and discovered that her GP was supportive and kind. This reinforced the pattern of frequent attendance, which she had earlier experienced with her own mother. Following the pregnancy with a threatened miscarriage, and then failure to be able to breast feed, she felt more depressed and first gave salt to the baby.

Interpretation – the therapist considered that when the mother had failed to breast feed the child, by a process of projection she perceived this as a personal deprivation and an attack on herself by the baby. Other influences also contributed to shaping the mother's behaviour, notably the family culture of excessive attendance at the doctor and in a secondary way the rewarding nature of the hospital environment in relieving her unpleasant mood-state.

Therapeutic relationship – the woman stated that she had found the therapist a consistent figure in an otherwise unreliable world.

Role of the father – although not included in the therapy sessions the father responded positively and moved from being a passive figure to becoming more involved in family life and an essential support to his wife.

Changes in therapy – there seemed reasonable collateral evidence for the following changes:

1 Further abuse had not occurred and the mother's care of all her children had not given rise to concern over a 15-month period.
2 There had been a cessation of her excessive attendances at the GP.
3 There were changes in her attitude to her religion. Less censorious and severe and more informed of her own humanity.
4 During therapy she was able to become more firm in her management of her father.
5 While never a demonstrative person, it was felt that she became generally warmer and more spontaneous socially.
6 Despite the pain of the events, the mother said that she was glad that she had been found out so that she could get the help she needed.

Individual psychotherapy as an inpatient

In the case described by Coombe (1995) the perpetrating mother had poisoned her two older children with salt. It is emphasized that the individual therapy was but one part of an extensive package of therapy delivered to the mother and child via group therapy for parents, family sessions and attendance of the child at the Children's Day Unit. The process commenced with a one-month inpatient assessment.

The findings during the assessment period included the observation of 'massive denial' of her own role in the loss of her two children who had been taken into the care of the local authority, with projection onto others and danger directed at them, notably the social worker. There was inability to bear frustration. The loss of her grandmother preceding the birth of her first child, and the birth had been difficult. There was an unsatisfactory relationship with the husband despite the marriage of several years. There were indicators that the woman could use the therapy being offered and therefore a treatment programme was implemented.

In the early phase of treatment (about four months) the mother developed an excessive sensitivity to separation from the daughter. This concerned the therapy team as it was thought it may indicate a very fragile state in which the mother feared (psychological) disintegration or collapse on separation from the daughter. Eventually she began to develop the rudiments of 'a capacity to feel concerned about her own mental state'. In the middle phase of about 12 months a group experience was added to the twice-weekly individual sessions. 'There was progressive and qualitative development in the capacity to experience loss.' In the later phase of about four months there was development of empathy for her daughter's position in relation to the imminent departure from the hospital. For over two years the consultant supervised therapy by other agencies and the report was that the child continued to develop well despite there being some ongoing difficulties for the mother of a relatively minor nature.

Family therapy

Black and Hollis (1996) describe the treatment of a family as outpatients. In their abstract they state that:

> with careful case selection and preparation, and with modifications to existing treatment approaches, we conclude that the generally poor prognosis for this condition may be improved. Safe rehabilitation of the child to the family can be a reasonable treatment goal in selected cases.

The authors reported this case in which treatment was successful in order to encourage paediatricians and child psychiatrists to seek treatment for such families. A summarized account of their paper is presented here.

The family included two boys, the index child referred to as Charlie (for the purpose of the paper) and a half-brother. Charlie was subjected to illness induction by his mother who had administered salt and Lactulose, and had tampered with a venous line. The child had lost half a kilogram in weight and suffered from immeasurable pain, thirst and distress with diarrhoea, vomiting and poor feeding, leading to lethargy and irritability. It emerged that the older half-brother had been investigated for chronic diarrhoea and had been taken to his GP on 69 occasions over four years. Charlie was discharged from hospital to live with the paternal grandparents where he was joined by his brother. Charlie's parents were allowed frequent, regular supervised access.

A notable feature was that, six months after the identification of the illness induction, the mother admitted the poisoning to her social worker. Subsequently she became depressed, lost weight and spoke of suicide. The mother improved with social work support and antidepressants prescribed by her GP. Recognising that the acknowledgement of the mother's behaviour represented a hopeful development, a referral was made to the psychiatric service to provide an opinion about the possibility of rehabilitation.

The assessment was carried out when Charlie was 14 months old with both parents and the two boys attending. Early on positive features were noted:

- The mother was able to acknowledge her actions in giving salt to her son, and identified life stresses at the time and her own intention to keep the child in hospital to get some sleep for herself.
- The husband was able to state that he had offered little support at the time.
- During the assessment the parents both took an active part in caring for the child and protecting him from danger.
- When observed from behind a screen, the mother was sensitively responding to the needs of the child.
- The wider family were continuing to be supportive.

As a result of the assessment it was decided to offer a course of therapeutic work, which the parents were eager to accept.

Following further assessment for psychotherapy a contract of ten sessions was offered to the couple and accepted. In summary, the therapy was brief and systemic, with cognitive and behavioural components. Three themes of the therapy are highlighted by the authors:

- Relationships – a family culture in at least three generations of women communicating distress by physical symptoms.
- Beliefs – two main beliefs appeared to be operating. First, that distress can be expressed and help elicited by the use of physical symptoms, and, second, that the mother feared that she would be criticized (by her husband, her mother and professionals) if she asked for help directly.
- Behaviour – the couple were able to improve their relationship and also developed a more maturely dependent relationship with the therapist whereby the couple were able to ask for help when necessary.

The outcome of the therapy was that after four more years both children were doing well with no significant symptoms or behavioural problems, and with no evidence of developmental delay or brain damage. The authors cautioned that some risk factors remained:

- The mother still tends to allocate inappropriate responsibility to the children.
- There is reluctance to engage in therapeutic work beyond a minimal level of behavioural change.
- There is a reluctance to consider the possibility of past illness induction in the older boy.

Sanders (1996) describes the successful treatment of a family in which the mother had fabricated and exaggerated illness in her children: twin boys. The management model employed included physician monitoring of all medical treatment throughout childhood together with narrative therapies. The author emphasizes that a mandatory aspect of any treatment plan will include the implementation of a 'safe' management plan.

Outcome of psychiatric intervention

Berg and Jones (1999) report on the outcome for 17 children from 16 families treated at the Park Hospital in Oxford. The mean follow-up interval was 27 months. Most of the children had been victims of fabrication at the severe end of the spectrum; 12 had been illness induction and one had included tampering with specimens. Information was obtained on the children and their carers from general practitioners, social workers or both; in addition 13 of the children and carers were interviewed.

At the Park Hospital the children and families were assessed and treated by a highly experienced multi-disciplinary child and family psychiatric team, whose work concentrates on child mal-treatment. Some admissions comprised in-depth assessments, whereas most examined the prospects for family re-unification. The treatment was a mixture of family work, individual treat-ment for parents using focal psychotherapeutic methods, includ-ing cognitive behaviour therapy, and brief focal psychotherapy combined with systemic family therapy. Infant–parent attach-ment theory is the cornerstone of the team's theoretical orien-tation.

The children were assessed in a number of areas:

- physical growth, neurological and social development
- an index of the child's tendency to somatize
- emotions and behaviour
- the social context – by interview with the main carer.

The carers were assessed in a number of areas:

- their perception of current stress
- psychological health and symptoms
- social adjustment.

The findings of the study

The Park team recommended rehabilitation for 13 children and alternative care for four. There was one instance of re-abuse by illness induction, which was observed quickly and no permanent harm was done. The child continued to reside with the birth father without the birth mother. All the children had grown normally. Six children showed mild developmental delays.

Most of the carers considered their children to be healthy at follow-up. For five children the perspective of the mother dif-fered from that of the GP. In four cases the mother had been exaggerating symptoms, which is of particular interest given the history of fabrication. In none of these were symptoms fabricated;

nevertheless in three of these cases there had been excessive attendance at the GP and excessive health concerns had caused problems for the GP and health visitor. In the fifth case the GP had been more concerned than the mother about her daughter's eczema.

Two children showed evidence of mild disturbance on the behaviour checklist but not severe enough to consider psychiatric referral.

Five of the carers showed evidence of psychological disturbance on examination of their mental states. Three showed signs of anxiety and mild depression and two were preoccupied with minor physical ailments. Five carers scored abnormally high on the parenting stress index. In all but one of the families treated there was retrospective insight by the main carer that she had originally harmed her child. One mother had no insight and the authors were concerned about her mental health although her child was in good health and no problems were evident.

Persistent concerns about the children were rated by the authors as serious concerns (two families/three children), mild concerns (five families) and no concerns (nine families) – the number of families placed in each category are indicated in brackets. One of the children for whom serious concerns were expressed had been a victim of illness induction by dilution of milk. Following work at the Park the child had been re-united with the mother at the age of two years. His mother remarried and had two further children. At the follow-up she described the boy as 'hyperactive, aggressive and psychologically disturbed'. She perceived him to be different to his siblings and described a poor attachment to him. The mother suspected that the boy had speech problems and anaemia and had contacted both her GP and health visitor. The woman had many health complaints herself, including episodes of fainting, anaemia and backache. For the latter she was attempting to claim compensation. The woman showed limited insight into the admission to the Park.

The child was over-familiar with the researcher. He appeared anxious and insecure in the attachment to his mother. There were no other problems in his development identified. The GP found the frequent attendance unacceptable and was considering removing her from his list. Notably the family had not received continued psychological help or social casework.

The authors concluded that family reunification is feasible for certain cases, but long-term follow-up is necessary to ensure the child's safety and to identify deterioration in the parents' mental health. The outcome for reunited children compared well with reported untreated cases.

References

Berg B, Jones DPH. Outcome of psychiatric intervention in factitious illness by proxy (Munchausen's syndrome by proxy). *Archives of Disease in Childhood.* 1999; **81**: 465–72.

Black D, Hollis P. Treatment of a case of factitious illness by proxy. *Clinical Child Psychology and Psychiatry.* 1996; **1**: 89–98.

Coombe P. The inpatient psychotherapy of a mother and child at the Cassel Hospital: a case of Munchausen's Syndrome by Proxy. *British J Psychotherapy.* 1995; **12**: 195–207.

Nicol AR, Eccles M. Psychotherapy for Munchausen syndrome by proxy. *Archives of Disease in Childhood.* 1985; **60**(4): 344–8.

Sanders MJ. Narrative family treatment of Munchausen by proxy: a successful case. *Families, Systems and Health.* 1996; **14**(3): 315–29.

Further reading

Bluglass K. Treatment of perpetrators. In: Adshead G, Brooke D, editors. *Munchausen's Syndrome by Proxy: current issues in assessment, treatment and research.* London: Imperial College Press; 2001.

Brooks D, Adshead G. Current challenges in the management of perpetrators. In: Adshead G, Brooke D, editors. *Munchausen's Syndrome by Proxy: current issues in assessment, treatment and research.* London: Imperial College Press; 2001.

Gray JA, Bentovim A, Milla P. The treatment of children and their families where induced illness has been identified. In: Horwath J, Lawson B, editors. *Trust Betrayed? Munchausen syndrome by proxy, inter-agency child protection and partnership with families.* London: National Children's Bureau; 1995.

Jones DPH, Byrne G, Newbould C. Management, treatment and outcomes. In: Eminson M, Postlethwaite RJ, editors. *Munchausen Syndrome by Proxy Abuse: a practical approach.* Oxford: Butterworth Heinemann; 2000. Out of print but pdf available on *Incredibly Caring.* Oxford: Radcliffe Publishing; 2007.

Mitchell I. Treatment and outcome for victims. In: Adshead G, Brooke D, editors. *Munchausen's Syndrome by Proxy: current issues in assessment, treatment and research.* London: Imperial College Press; 2001.

Parnell TF, Day DO. *Munchausen Syndrome by Proxy: misunderstood child abuse.* Thousand Oaks: Sage; 1998. Part II (Chapters 6 to 12): Intervention with the perpetrator and family.

Chapter 8

Incidence and knowledge of FII

Section headings
How common, or rare, is FII?
A study in New Zealand
A survey of paediatricians in the USA
What do professionals know about FII?
Effects on paediatric nursing staff
A model of the staff's reactions
KEY WORDS/PHRASES
Epidemiology of FII
Annual incidence
Professionals' knowledge
How to document behaviour
Staff support

How common, or rare, is FII?

The epidemiology of FII was investigated in the UK and Ireland when paediatricians carried out a two-year prospective study with notification being made to the British Paediatric Association Surveillance Unit (McClure *et al.*, 1996). Cases of FII (MSP), together with non-accidental poisoning and non-accidental suffocation, were included. The time interval was two years, from September 1992 to August 1994. The reporting criterion was if a formal child protection case conference had been held to discuss any of the above problems.

One hundred and twenty-eight cases were identified: 55 were FII alone, 15 poisoning and 15 suffocation, and 43 suffered more than one type of abuse. Most of the child victims were under five years of age. In 42% of the families a sibling had suffered from some form of abuse. The annual incidence calculated from these findings was at least 0.5/100,000 in children aged less than 16, and at least 2.8/100,000 for children aged less than one year. The number of girl and boy victims was approximately equal (60 and 68, respectively). In respect of the question as to whether all cases were actually reported to the research team, the variation in incidence by a factor of 7 between two of the Health Authorities (administrative regions) suggests that this was not the case. By inference this also suggests that the actual incidence was probably higher than that recorded by the researchers.

The researchers reported that 92 cases (72%) first presented as paediatric emergencies. The presentation involved fabricated signs or interference with test results in 21 cases. Fifty-three cases involved illness induction. The co-occurrence of suffocation and non-accidental poisoning, as methods of illness induction, in the context of fabrication of illness was noted by the researchers. Because of this co-occurrence, and probably in respect of the relative rarity of all three situations, the study included examples of suffocation and non-accidental poisoning even when not associated with fabrication of illness. The severity of the abuse was notable; eight index children died either as result of poisoning or suffocation, 15 more children required treatment in paediatric intensive care, another 45 children suffered major physical illness and 31 minor physical illnesses. In this study, which focused on the short term, the psychological harm was not assessed.

The paediatricians reporting to the researchers had been asked to rate their certainty of the diagnosis of FII: 109 paediatricians (85%) rated the probability of their diagnosis to be correct as greater than 90%. The mother was the sole perpetrator in 109 cases (85%). The father was implicated alone on six occasions. The remainder were: in one case a grandfather, in one case a boyfriend of the mother, in 11 cases the perpetrator remained uncertain.

The situation with regard to siblings of the index children was reported and indicates that a high level of attention and concern should be given to siblings when FII is identified. Eighty-three of 128 index children had at least one sibling. Fifteen index children had a sibling who had died previously (18 siblings). In 34 families a sibling had suffered from abuse previously. The incidence of types of abuse was: FII 17, suffocation 5, poisoning 5, physical 5 and neglect 5.

The survey is important in providing, for the first time, a figure for the incidence of FII across the UK and Republic of Ireland with implications for identification, training of staff and the provision of services (and therefore implications for a number of organizations including: hospitals, primary care trusts, social services, education authorities, and legal services). There has been no update of this study, which is now more than 10 years old, and therefore it is not known if the annual incidence of FII has changed.

A study in New Zealand

A study of the epidemiology of FII, carried out in a manner similar to the McClure *et al.* (1996) study above, was carried out amongst paediatricians in New Zealand during 1999 (Denny *et al.*, 2001). The response rate was good with 95% of practising paediatricians responding. Eighteen cases of FII were identified during the 12-month period, giving an annual incidence of 200/100,000 children aged less than 16 years old. When cases were excluded that had not been referred to child protection agencies the figure was 1.2/100,000. This latter figure is three times the incidence reported by McClure *et al.* in the UK (as the rate of FII only in the McClure *et al.* study is 0.4/100,000).

A survey of paediatricians in the USA

A survey of paediatric neurologists and gastroenterologists was carried out in spring 1991. Eight hundred and seventy of the former and 388 of the latter were mailed; 190 and 126 responded, 22% and 32% respectively. The two groups combined reported a total of 465 cases of FII, of which 273 were confirmed and 192 seriously suspected. A sibling was believed to be involved in 120 (25.8%) of the 465 possible cases. The survey showed an average length of time before diagnosis to be more than a year in 19% and more than six months in 33% (Schreier and Libow, 1993).

What do professionals know about FII?

Kaufman *et al.* (1989) from Columbus, Ohio, USA, surveyed 86 professionals from medicine, social services and legal agencies about their knowledge of FII. Professionals from medical and hospital-based settings were three times as likely to have heard of MSP (FII) than those employed by community services.

Effects on paediatric nursing staff

Blix and Brack (1988) from Indiana, USA, carried out a survey of 20 nursing staff from a ward one to two weeks after a case of FII had been discharged from the ward. Questionnaires were completed anonymously (and this aspect was emphasized to the nurses). Supervising physicians and residents declined to take part in the study.

The 17-month-old child victim of FII had been presented with recurrent urinary tract infections, which (it was initially assumed) accounted for the recurrent low-grade fevers, weight loss, recurrent vomiting and developmental delays. A central line was placed (in a major vein) in order for her to receive nutrition intravenously. The infections continued and did not cease until the central line was removed and antibiotics had been given by injections into muscle that numbered 21 per day. The child began to make gains when the parents were restricted and supervised in their visits to the child. Following multiple investigations the conclusion of the physicians was that the mother had been deliberately introducing infective materials (enteric in origin: i.e. sourced from faeces) into the tube feeding the central line.

The results of the survey indicated that only 10% of the nurses had previously encountered a case of FII. Seventy-five per cent said that they were not professionally prepared and 80% felt emotionally unprepared. Many felt unclear about their role including how to *document behaviour* of the parents. The majority of the nurses described difficulty in accepting that fabrication and illness induction was occurring and even when intellectually accepting the diagnosis of FII they felt emotionally that it was difficult to accept. The emotions experienced included feeling 'sickened and repelled by the idea' in one quarter and many indicated angry feelings.

With regard to the effect on future practice, 65% indicated that their views on patients and their families had been affected, and 40% thought there would be an effect on future relationships with patients and families. The issue was raised as to when the physician might have discussed the possibility of FII with all the nursing staff. The usefulness of staff unity and support was listed as helping the staff to deal with such a situation. They advised other professionals when facing a similar situation of the need for *staff support* and the discussion of negative feelings, that such reactions are to be expected and can be dealt with effectively by staff discussions, group support and self-acceptance. The need for more information about the case was mentioned by more than one quarter of the staff. Finally one nurse warned of the splitting that can occur between staff members and between staff groups as a consequence of the behaviour and psychological functioning of the fabricating parent. (*See* Box 8.1.)

Box 8.1   A model of the staff's reactions to the case (of FII)

1 Initial interactions with suspected parent:
   a Parent is perceived as loving, concerned, and caring.
   b Some of the staff feel 'close' to parents.
2 Immediate effects on learning of suspected diagnosis:
   a Intense feelings of shock, disbelief, and denial, accompanied in many cases by nausea and repulsion.
   b Need for more information and definition of nursing role that is satisfied by library research, in-services, etc.
3 Subsequent short-term effects:
   a Acceptance of diagnosis as correct, at least on intellectual level.
   b Increased vigilance and monitoring of parent–child interactions of all parents.
   c Among minority of staff a tendency to distrust parents in general.
4 Hypothesized long-term effects:
   a Education about the disease and potentially increased ability to recognize further cases.
   b Among at least a few staff members continued increased vigilance and monitoring of parent–child interactions.
   c Among a small minority of staff members a continued tendency to distrust parents.

(From Blix and Brack, 1988.)

References

Blix S, Brack G. The effects of a suspected case of Munchausen's syndrome by proxy on a pediatric nursing staff. *General Hospital Psychiatry*. 1988; 10: 402–9.

Denny SJ, Grant CC, Pinnock R. Epidemiology of Munchausen syndrome by proxy in New Zealand. *J Paediatrics and Child Health*. 2001; 37: 240–3.

Kaufman KL, Coury D, Pickrel E, McCleery J. Munchausen syndrome by proxy: a survey of professionals' knowledge. *Child Abuse and Neglect.* 1989; 13: 141–7.

McClure RJ, Davis PM, Meadow SR, Sibert JR. Epidemiology of Munchausen syndrome by proxy, non-accidental poisoning, and non-accidental suffocation. *Archives of Disease in Childhood.* 1996; 75: 57–61.

Schreier HA, Libow JA. Munchausen syndrome by proxy: diagnosis and prevalence. *American Journal of Orthopsychiatry.* 1993; 63: 318–21.

Further reading

Bradley S. The child first and always? *Paediatric Nursing.* 1998; 10: 23–6.

Brown ML. Dilemmas facing nurses who care for Munchausen syndrome by proxy patients. *Pediatric Nursing.* 1997; 23: 416–18.

Middleton C. Nursing issues related to Munchausen syndrome by proxy. In: Horwath J, Lawson B, editors. *Trust Betrayed? Munchausen syndrome by proxy, inter-agency child protection and partnership with families.* London: National Children's Bureau; 1995.

Chapter 9

Prevention of FII

Section headings
Strategies for prevention
  Universal prevention
  Targeted prevention
  Specialist prevention
KEY WORDS/PHRASES
Reduce impact of fabricating behaviours
Psychiatric disorder
Increased risk
Primary healthcare services
Risk factors
Progression to FII
Susceptible mother
Protective factors
Exaggeration
Early safeguarding and treatment interventions

Strategies for prevention

The core aim of preventative intervention is to prevent/min-imize/reduce the impact of the fabricating behaviour, and any associated problems, on parents and their children. This aim varies only a little from that regarding the work that may be carried out to reduce the impact of parental mental illness upon children as described in *Crossing Bridges* (Falkov, 1998). Since psychiatric disorders (including personality disorder and psychi-atric illness) have been demonstrated to be common in the fabricator, most if not all of the detail of the *Crossing Bridges* reader is relevant to FII with its potential to lead to impairment of the development of the child, and the functioning of the parent. A suggested strategy for universal, targeted and specialist pre-vention of FII and its impact is set out in Box 9.1.

Box 9.1   A preventative strategy for FII

Universal prevention (response to evidence of recent existence of FII in society).

- Consideration of (hypothesized) contributing factors resulting from aspects of the organization of society in which FII has been reported, in particular local medical and social systems.
- Planning of services that are likely to reduce the occurrence of FII.
- Specific measures include the provision of effective social and health services for families, i.e. services for parents and their children throughout the life cycle.

Targeted prevention (response to evidence that certain families in society [parents and children] are at an increased risk of adverse impact of FII, including consideration of a higher incidence in certain health and social service areas/systems).

- Careful support and monitoring of 'mothers at risk' of FII as a consequence of suffering from particular psychiatric disorders; certain personality disorders, persistent and severe forms of somatization, repeated self-harm (especially when occurring in combination with each other and in combination with evidence of deceptive behaviour) and other severe psychiatric disorders, including post-natal depression, in combination with the above.
- Additional support from primary healthcare services when such women are about to start a family and from birth onwards.
- Identification of factors in the pregnancy and the early life of the child that may increase the risk of a progression to FII.
- Evidence of behaviours which could lead on to fabrication in a susceptible mother; frequent presentation at healthcare facilities and evidence of increasing (becoming unrealistic) worries about the health of the child, exaggeration about the health status of the child and

particularly increasing fantasy and making statements that are not objectively true.

- Children who may be showing general signs of unhappiness and stress, and perhaps specifically showing evidence of becoming involved in the exaggerations, fantasy and untruths about the state of their own health: becoming seriously preoccupied with health problems for which there is no objective evidence.

Specialist prevention (response to evidence that FII has occurred, or is strongly suspected).

- Provision of services that offer a broad assessment of risk and protective factors in the family in a context of childcare circumstances (*see* the Assessment Framework).
- Provision of health and social services that provide early safeguarding and treatment interventions for the mother and family.
- Assessment, treatment and rehabilitation of developmental and psychiatric disorder in the child.
- Promotion of strengths and protective factors in the family.

Whilst this Reader has focused primarily on secondary prevention, it is hoped that in the future more primary preventative work will be possible. We now have a substantial knowledge base specifically with regard to FII. This may be added to the existing wider knowledge base, which addresses the difficulties for professionals in working with the combination of treating parents' mental health problems and protecting/safeguarding children from harm.

What are now available in most local areas are **opportunities** for:

- improved planning
- education and training for professionals
- appropriate, balanced information for the public
- allocation of resources
- good communication between agencies and professionals: the promotion of effective networks.

As a result we hope that professionals working in this challenging area will:

- maintain an open mind about the possibility of FII, and that they
- are supported by their organizations to be in a position to offer interventions
- which are timely and appropriate to the level of need and risk, and that they will
- continue to look for preventative interventions which will offer an opportunity to prevent progression to a more serious form of the potentially harmful behaviours, and
- eventually for opportunities for (primary) prevention of FII.

Reference

Falkov A. *Crossing Bridges. Training resources for working with mentally ill parents and their children: Reader – for managers, practitioners and trainers*. Brighton: Pavilion Publishing, for the Department of Health; 1998.

Reference list

Full listing for all chapters of references and recommended further reading.

Ackerman NB, Strobel CT. Polle syndrome: chronic diarrhea in Munchausen's child. *Gastroenterology*. 1981; **81**(6): 1140–2.

Adcock M, White M. *Significant Harm: its management and outcome*, 2nd edition. Croydon: Significant Publications; 1998.

Adshead G, Bluglass K. A vicious circle: transgenerational attachment representations in a case of factitious illness by proxy. *Attachment and Human Development*. 2001; **3**(1): 77–95.

Alexander R, Smith W, Stevenson R. Serial Munchausen syndrome by proxy. *Pediatrics*. 1990; **86**(4): 581–5.

American Psychiatric Association. *Diagnostic and Statistical Manual of Mental Disorder (Fourth Edition) DSM-IV*. Washington DC: American Psychiatric Association; 1994.

Atoynatan TH, O'Reilly E, Loin L. Munchausen syndrome by proxy. *Child Psychiatry and Human Development*. 1988; **19**(1): 3–13.

Bass C, Murphy M. Somatoform and personality disorders: syndromal co-morbidity and overlapping developmental pathways. *J Psychosomatic Research*. 1995; **39**: 403–27.

Belsky J. Child maltreatment: an ecological integration. *American Psychologist*. 1980; **35**: 320–35.

Bentovim A. A 20-year overview. In: Adshead G, Brooke D, editors. *Munchausen's Syndrome by Proxy. Current issues in assessment, treatment and research*. London: Imperial College Press; 2001.

Berg B, Jones DPH. Outcome of psychiatric intervention in factitious illness by proxy (Munchausen's syndrome by proxy). *Archives of Disease in Childhood*. 1999; **81**: 465–72.

Black D. The extended Munchausen syndrome: a family case. *British Journal of Psychiatry*. 1981; **138**: 466–9.

Black D, Hollis P. Treatment of a case of factitious illness by proxy. *Clinical Child Psychology and Psychiatry*. 1996; **1**: 89–98.

Blix S, Brack G. The effects of a suspected case of Munchausen's syndrome by proxy on a pediatric nursing staff. *General Hospital Psychiatry*. 1988; **10**: 402–9.

Bluglass K. Treatment of perpetrators. In: Adshead G, Brooke D, editors. *Munchausen's Syndrome by Proxy. Current issues in assessment, treatment and research*. London: Imperial College Press; 2001.

Bools CN, Neale BA, Meadow SR. Co-morbidity associated with fabricated illness (Munchausen syndrome by proxy). *Archives of Disease in Childhood*. 1992; **67**: 77–9.

Bools CN, Neale BA, Meadow SR. Follow up of victims of fabricated illness (Munchausen Syndrome by Proxy). *Archives of Disease in Childhood*. 1993; **69**: 625–30.

Bools CN, Neale BA, Meadow SR. Munchausen Syndrome by Proxy: a study of psychopathology. *Child Abuse and Neglect*. 1994; **18**: 773–88.

Bowlby J. *Attachment and Loss. Vol. 1 Attachment*. London: Hogarth Press and the Institute of Psychoanalysis; 1969.

Bourchier D. Bleeding ears: case report of Munchausen syndrome by proxy. *Australian Paediatric Journal*. 1983; **19**(4): 256–7.

Boyce WT. The vulnerable child: new evidence, new approaches. *Advanced Paediatrics*. 1992; **39**: 1–33.

Bradley S. The child first and always? *Paediatric Nursing*. 1998; **10**: 23–6.

Brooks D, Adshead G. Current challenges in the management of perpetrators. In: Adshead G, Brooke D, editors. *Munchausen's Syndrome by Proxy. Current issues in assessment, treatment and research*. London: Imperial College Press; 2001.

Brown ML. Dilemmas facing nurses who care for Munchausen syndrome by proxy patients. *Pediatric Nursing*. 1997; **23**: 416–18.

Bryk M, Siegel PT. My mother caused my illness: the story of a survivor of Munchausen by Proxy Syndrome. *Pediatrics*. 1997; **100**: 1–7.

Chan DA, Salcedo JR, Atkins DM, Ruley EJ. Munchausen syndrome by proxy: a review and case study. *Journal of Pediatric Psychology*. 1986; **11**(1): 71–80.

Coombe P. The Inpatient Psychotherapy of a Mother and Child at the Cassel Hospital: A Case of Munchausen's Syndrome by Proxy. *British J Psychotherapy*. 1995; **12**: 195–207.

Craig TK, Boardman AP, Mills K, Daly-Jones O, Drake H. The south London somatisation study. I: Longitudinal course and the influence of early life experience. *British J Psychiatry*. 1993; **163**: 579–88.

Craig TK, Drake H, Mills K, Boardman AP. The south London somatisation study. II: Influence of stressful life events, and secondary gain. *British J Psychiatry*. 1994; **165**: 248–58.

Croft RD, Jervis M. Munchausen's syndrome in a 4-year-old. *Archives of Disease in Childhood*. 1989; **64**: 740–1.

Davis P, McClure RJ, Rolfe K, Chessman N, Pearson S, Sibert JR, Meadow R. Procedures, placement, and risks of further abuse after Munchausen Syndrome by Proxy, non-accidental poisoning and non-accidental suffocation. *Archives of Disease in Childhood*. 1998; **78**: 217–21.

Denny SJ, Grant CC, Pinnock R. Epidemiology of Munchausen syndrome by proxy in New Zealand. *J Paediatrics and Child Health*. 2001; **37**: 240–3.

Department of Health. *Assessing Children's Needs and Circumstances: the impact of the Assesment Framework*. London, Department of Health Publications; 2003.

Department of Health, Department for Education and Employment and the Home Office. *Framework for the Assessment of Children in Need and Their Families*. London: The Stationery Office; 2000.

Department of Health, Home Office, Department for Education and Skills, Welsh Assembly Government. *Safeguarding Children in Whom Illness is Fabricated or Induced*. London: Department of Health, Home Office, Department for Education and Skills, Welsh Assembly Government; August 2002. www.dfes.gov.uk/qualityprotects/info/publications/childprot.shtml

Dershewitz R, Vestal B, Maclaren NK, Cornblath M. Transient hepatomegaly and hypoglycemia: a consequence of malicious insulin administration. *American Journal of Diseases of Children.* 1976; **130**: 998–9.

Dine MS, McGovern ME. Intentional poisoning of children – an overlooked category of child abuse: report of seven cases and review of the literature. *Pediatrics.* 1982; **70**(1): 32–5.

Eisendrath SJ. Factitious illness: a clarification. *Psychosomatics.* 1984; **25**: 110–17.

Eminson DM, Postlethwaite RJ. Factitious illness: recognition and management. *Archives of Disease in Childhood.* 1992; **67**: 1510–16.

Eminson M. Munchausen syndrome by proxy – an introduction. In: Eminson M, Postlethwaite RJ, editors. *Munchausen Syndrome by Proxy Abuse: a practical approach.* Oxford: Butterworth Heinemann; 2000. Out of print but pdf available on *Incredibly Caring.* Oxford: Radcliffe Publishing; 2007.

Epstein MA, Markowitz RL, Gallo DM, Holmes JW, Gryboski JD. Munchausen syndrome by proxy: considerations in diagnosis and confirmation by video surveillance. *Pediatrics.* 1987; **80**(2): 220–4.

Erickson MF, Egeland B. Child neglect. In: Briere J, Berliner L, Bulkley JA, Jenny C, Reid T, editors. *The APSAC Handbook on Child Maltreatment.* Thousand Oaks, California: Sage; 1996.

Falkov A. *Crossing Bridges. Training resources for working with mentally ill parents and their children. Reader – for managers, practitioners and trainers.* Brighton: Pavilion Publishing, for the Department of Health; 1998.

Feldman KW, Christopher DM, Opheim KB. Munchausen syndrome/bulimia by proxy: ipecac as a toxin in child abuse. *Child Abuse and Neglect.* 1989; **13**: 257–61.

Fialkov MJ. Peregrination in the problem pediatric patient: the pediatric Munchhausen syndrome? *Clinical Pediatrics.* 1984; **23**(10): 571–5.

Fisher GC, Mitchell I, Murdoch D. Munchausen's syndrome by proxy. The question of psychiatric illness in a child. *British Journal of Psychiatry.* 1993; **162**: 701–3.

Fleisher D, Ament ME. Diarrhea, red diapers, and child abuse. *Clinical Pediatrics.* 1977; **17**(9): 820–4.

Freeland H, Foley, S. The management of polarisation in Munchausen syndrome by proxy. In: Calvert G, Ford A, Parkinson P, editors. *The Practice of Child Protection: Australian approaches.* Sydney: Hale and Iremonger; 1992.

Geelhoed GC, Pemberton PJ. SIDS, seizures or 'sophageal reflux? Another manifestation of Munchausen syndrome by proxy. *Medical Journal of Australia.* 1985; **143**(8): 357–8.

Gibbons J, Gallagher B, Bell C, Gordon D. *Development After Physical Abuse in Early Childhood.* London: HMSO; 1995.

Gill D, Bass C. Somatoform and dissociative disorders: assessment and treatment. *Advances in Psychiatric Treatment.* 1997; **3**: 9–16.

Godding V, Kruth M. Compliance with treatment in asthma and Munchausen syndrome by proxy. *Archives of Disease in Childhood.* 1991; **66**: 956–60.

Gray J. The social work role in Munchausen syndrome by proxy. In: Adshead G, Brooke D, editors. *Munchausen's Syndrome by Proxy. Current issues in assessment, treatment and research*. London: Imperial College Press; 2001.

Gray J, Bentovim A. Illness induction syndrome: paper I – a series of 41 children from 37 families identified at the Great Ormond Street Hospital for Children NHS Trust. *Child Abuse and Neglect*. 1996; **20**: 655–73.

Gray JA, Bentovim A, Milla P. The treatment of children and their families where induced illness has been identified. In: Horwath J, Lawson B, editors. *Trust Betrayed? Munchausen syndrome by proxy, inter-agency child protection and partnership with families*. London: National Children's Bureau; 1995.

Green M, Solnit AJ. Reactions to the loss of a child: A vulnerable child syndrome. *Pediatrics*. 1964; **34**: 58–66.

Green M. Vulnerable child syndrome and its variants. *Pediatrics in Review*. 1986; **8**(3): 75–80.

Gregory J. *Sickened. The true story of a lost childhood*. London: Arrow Books; 2004.

Griffith JL. The family systems of Munchausen syndrome by proxy. *Family Process*. 1988; **27**: 423–37.

Guandolo VL. Munchausen syndrome by proxy: an outpatient challenge. *Pediatrics*. 1985; **75**(3): 526–30.

Hardwick P. Health beliefs and myths in child and adolescent practice. *Clinical Child Psychology Psychiatry*. 1998; **3**: 87–102.

Hardwick PJ. Families' medical myths. *Journal of Family Therapy*. 1989; **11**: 3–27.

Henderson S. Care-eliciting behaviour in man. *J Nervous and Mental Disease*. 1974; **159**: 172–81.

HM Government. *Working Together to Safeguard Children: a guide for interagency working to safeguard and promote the welfare of children*. London: The Stationery Office; 2006.

HM Government. *Safeguarding Children in Whom Illness is Fabricated or Induced*. London: Department for Education and Skills; 2007. www.everychildmatters. gov.uk/safeguarding

Hodge D, Schwartz W, Sargent J, Bodurtha J, Starr S. The bacteriologically battered baby: another case of Munchausen syndrome by proxy. *Annals of Emergency Medicine*. 1982; **11**(4): 205–7.

Horwath J. Inter-agency practice in suspected cases of Munchausen syndrome by proxy (Fictitious illness by proxy): dilemmas for professionals. *Child and Family Social Work*. 1999; **4**: 109–18.

Horwath J. Developing good practice in cases of fabricated and induced illness by carers: new guidance and training implications. *Child Abuse Review*. 2003; **12**: 58–63.

Horwath J, Lawson B, editors. *Trust Betrayed? Munchausen syndrome by proxy, inter-agency child protection and partnership with families*. London: National Children's Bureau; 1995.

Hosch IA. Munchausen syndrome by proxy. *American Journal of Maternal Child Nursing*. 1987; **12**(1): 48–52.

Jones DPH. Dermatitis artefacta in mother and baby as child abuse. *British Journal of Psychiatry*. 1983; **143**: 199–200.

Jones DPH, Byrne G, Newbould C. Management, treatment and outcomes. In: Eminson M, Postlethwaite RJ, editors. *Munchausen Syndrome by Proxy Abuse: a practical approach*. Oxford: Butterworth Heinemann; 2000. Out of print but pdf available on *Incredibly Caring*. Oxford: Radcliffe Publishing; 2007.

Jones JG, Butler HL, Hamilton B, Perdue JD, Stern HP, Woody RC. Munchausen syndrome by proxy. *Child Abuse and Neglect*. 1986; 10: 33–40.

Jureidini J. Obstetric Factitious Disorder and Munchausen syndrome by proxy. *Journal of Nervous and Mental Disease*. 1993; 181: 135–7.

Kaufman KL, Coury D, Pickrel E, McCleery J. Munchausen syndrome by proxy: a survey of professionals' knowledge. *Child Abuse and Neglect*. 1989; 13: 141–7.

Kessler RW. Personal communication (1980). Quoted by Waller (1983).

Kleinman A, Kleinman J. Somatisation: the interconnections in Chinese society among culture, depressive experiences, and the meanings of pain. In: Kleinman A, Good B, editors. *Culture and Depression*. Berkeley, Los Angeles: University of California; 1985.

Koch C, Hoiby N. Severe child abuse presenting as polymicrobial bacteremia. *Acta Paediatrica Scandinavica*. 1988; 77: 940–3.

Kravitz RM, Wilmott RW. Munchausen syndrome by proxy presenting as factitious apnea. *Clinical Pediatrics*. 1990; 29: 587–92.

Krener P. Factitious disorders and the psychosomatic continuum in children. *Current Opinion in Pediatrics*. 1994; 6: 418–22.

Krener P, Adelman R. Parent salvage and parent sabotage in the care of chronically ill children. *American Journal of Diseases of Children*. 1988; 142(9): 945–51.

Kurlandsky I, Lukoff JY, Zinkham WH, Brody JP, Kessler RW. Munchausen syndrome by proxy: definition of factitious bleeding by 51Cr labeling of erythrocytes. *Pediatrics*. 1979; 63(2): 228–31.

Lee DA. Munchausen syndrome by proxy in twins. *Archives of Disease in Childhood*. 1979; 54(8): 646–7.

Livingston R. Maternal somatization disorder and Munchausen syndrome by proxy. *Psychosomatics*. 1987; 28(4): 213–15.

Loader P, Kelly C. Munchausen Syndrome by Proxy: a narrative approach to explanation. *Clinical Child Psychology and Psychiatry*. 1996; 1: 353–63.

Lynch MA, Roberts J. *Consequences of Child Abuse*. London: Academic Press; 1982.

Makar AF, Squier PJ. Munchausen syndrome by proxy: father as perpetrator. *Pediatrics*. 1990; 85(3): 370–3.

Malatack JJ, Wiener ES, Gartner JC, Zitelli BJ, Brunetti E. Munchausen syndrome by proxy: a new complication of central venous catheterization. *Pediatrics*. 1985; 75(3): 523–5.

Masterson J, Dunworth R, Williams N. Extreme illness exaggeration in pediatric patients: a variant of Munchausen's by proxy? *American Journal of Orthopsychiatry*. 1988; 58(2): 188–95.

McClure RJ, Davis PM, Meadow SR, Sibert JR. Epidemiology of Munchausen syndrome by proxy, non-accidental poisoning, and non-accidental suffocation. *Archives of Disease in Childhood*. 1996; 75: 57–61.

McGuire TL, Feldman KW. Psychologic morbidity of children subjected to Munchausen syndrome by proxy. *Pediatrics*. 1989; **83**(2): 289–92.

Meadow R. Munchausen syndrome by proxy. *Archives of Disease in Childhood*. 1982; **57**(2): 92–8.

Mechanic D. The concept of illness behaviour. *J Chronic Disease*. 1962; **15**:189–94.

Mechanic D. The influence of mothers on their children's health attitudes and behavior. *Pediatrics*. 1964; **33**: 444–53.

Mechanic D. The concept of illness behaviour: culture, situation and personal predisposition. *Psychological Medicine*. 1986; **16**: 1–7.

Mehl AL, Coble L, Johnson S. Munchausen syndrome by proxy: A family affair. *Child Abuse and Neglect*. 1990; **14**: 577–85.

Middleton C. Nursing issues related to Munchausen syndrome by proxy. In: Horwath J, Lawson B, editors. *Trust Betrayed? Munchausen syndrome by proxy, inter-agency child protection and partnership with families*. London: National Children's Bureau; 1995.

Miller S. Family court: matter of Jessica Z. *New York Law Journal*. 1987; 3 March: 13.

Mitchell I. Treatment and outcome for victims. In: Adshead G, Brooke D, editors. *Munchausen's Syndrome by Proxy. Current issues in assessment, treatment and research*. London: Imperial College Press; 2001.

Morris B. Child abuse manifested as factitious apnea. *Southern Medical Journal*. 1985; **78**: 1013–14.

Morrison T. *Staff Supervision in Social Care. Making a real difference for staff and service users*. Brighton: Pavilion; 2001.

Nading JH, Duval-Arnould B. Factitious diabetes mellitus confirmed by ascorbic acid. *Archives of Disease in Childhood*. 1984; **59**(2): 166–7.

Neale B, Bools C, Meadow R. Problems in the assessment and management of Munchausen syndrome by proxy abuse. *Children and Society*. 1991; **5**: 324–33.

Nicol AR, Eccles M. Psychotherapy for Munchausen syndrome by proxy. *Archives of Disease in Childhood*. 1985; **60**(4): 344–8.

Orenstein DM, Wasserman AL. Munchausen syndrome by proxy simulating cystic fibrosis. *Pediatrics*. 1986; **78**(4): 621–4.

Osborne JP. Non-accidental poisoning and child abuse. *British Medical Journal*. 1976; **May 15**: 1211.

Outwater KM, Lipnick RN, Luban NLC, Ravenscroft K, Ruley EJ. Factitious hematuria: diagnosis by minor blood group typing. *Journal of Pediatrics*. 1981; **98**(1): 95–7.

Palmer AJ, Yoshimura GJ. Munchausen syndrome by proxy. *J American Academy Child and Adolescent Psychiatry*. 1984; **23**(4): 503–8.

Parnell TF, Day DO, editors. *Munchausen Syndrome by Proxy: misunderstood child abuse*. Thousand Oaks: Sage; 1998. Part II (Chapters 6 to 12): Intervention with the perpetrator and family.

Parrish M, Perman J. Munchausen syndrome by proxy: some practice implications for social workers. *Child and Adolescent Social Work Journal*. 2004; **21**: 137–54.

Parsons T. *The Social System*. New York: The Free Press; 1951.

Pearce D, Bools C. The child protection process. In: Eminson M, Postlethwaite RJ, editors. *Munchausen Syndrome by Proxy Abuse: a practical approach*. Oxford: Butterworth Heinemann; 2000. Out of print but pdf available on *Incredibly Caring*. Oxford: Radcliffe Publishing; 2007.

Pickford E, Buchanan N, McLaughlan S. Munchausen syndrome by proxy: a family anthology. *Medical Journal of Australia*. 1988; **148**(12): 646–50.

Pilowsky I. Abnormal illness behaviour. *British Journal of Medical Psychology*. 1969; **42**: 347–51.

Pilowsky I. Illness behaviour and neuroses. *Current Opinion in Psychiatry*. 1989; **2**: 217–24.

Pizzey S. The role of the guardian ad litem. In: Adshead G, Brooke D, editors. *Munchausen's Syndrome by Proxy. Current issues in assessment, treatment and research*. London: Imperial College Press; 2001.

Richardson GF. Munchausen syndrome by proxy. *American Family Physician*. 1987; **36**(1): 119–23.

Rogers D, Tripp J, Bentovim A, Robinson A, Berry D, Goulding R. Non-accidental poisoning: an extended syndrome of child abuse. *British Medical Journal*. 1976; **1**: 793–6.

Rosen CL, Frost JD, Bricker T, Tarnow JD, Gillette PC, Dunlavy S. Two siblings with recurrent cardiorespiratory arrest: Munchausen syndrome by proxy or child abuse? *Pediatrics*. 1983; **71**(5): 715–20.

Rosen CL, Frost JD, Glaze DG. Child abuse and recurrent infant apnea. *Journal of Pediatrics*. 1986; **109**(6): 1065–7.

Rosenberg DA. Web of deceit: a literature review of Munchausen syndrome by proxy. *Child Abuse and Neglect*. 1987; **11**(4): 547–63.

Rosenberg D. Munchausen Syndrome by Proxy: medical diagnostic criteria. *Child Abuse and Neglect*. 2003; **27**(4): 421–30.

Roth D. How 'mild' is mild Munchausen syndrome by proxy? *Israel Journal of Psychiatry and Related Science*. 1990; **27**: 160–7.

Royal College of Paediatrics and Child Health. *Fabricated or Induced Illness by Carers*. London: Royal College of Paediatrics and Child Health; February 2002. www.rcpch.ac.uk

Samuels MP, McClaughlin W, Jacobson RR, Poets CF, Southall DP. Fourteen cases of imposed upper airway obstruction. *Archives of Disease in Childhood*. 1992; **67**: 162–70.

Sanders MJ. Symptom coaching: factitious disorder by proxy with older children. *Clinical Psychology Review*. 1995; **15**: 423–42.

Sanders MJ. Narrative family treatment of Munchausen by proxy: a successful case. *Families, Systems and Health*. 1996; **14**(3): 315–29.

Sanders MJ. Hospital protocol for the evaluation of Munchausen syndrome by proxy. *Clinical Child Psychology and Psychiatry*. 1995; **4**: 379–91.

Schreier HA, Libow JA. Munchausen syndrome by proxy: diagnosis and prevalence. *American Journal of Orthopsychiatry*. 1993; **63**: 318–21.

Sheridan MS. The deceit continues; an updated literature review of Munchausen Syndrome by Proxy. *Child Abuse and Neglect*. 2003; **27**(4): 431–51.

Shnaps Y, Frand M, Rotem Y, Tirosh M. The chemically abused child. *Pediatrics*. 1981; **61**(1): 119–21.

Simms A. *Symptoms in the Mind: an introduction to descriptive psychopathology.* London: Baillière Tindall; 1988.

Sneed RC, Bell RF. The dauphin of Munchausen: factitious passage of renal stones in a child. *Pediatrics.* 1976; **58:** 127–30.

Stankler L. Factitious skin lesions in a mother and two sons. *British Journal of Dermatology.* 1977; **97:** 217–19.

Stevenson RD, Alexander R. Munchausen syndrome by proxy presenting as a developmental disability. *Developmental and Behavioral Pediatrics.* 1990; **11:** 262–4.

Stone FB. Munchausen by proxy syndrome: An unusual form of child abuse. *Social Casework.* 1989; **April:** 243–6.

Taylor DC. Outlandish Factitious Illness. In: David TJ, editor. *Recent Advances in Paediatrics. Number 10.* Edinburgh: Churchill Livingstone; 1992, Chapter 4, pp 63–76.

Underdown A, Birks E. *Professional Briefing Paper. Faltering Growth: taking the failure out of failure to thrive.* London: The Children's Society; date unknown.

Verity CM, Winckworth C, Burman D, Stevens D, White RJ. Polle syndrome: children of Munchausen. *British Medical Journal.* 1979; **2**(6187): 422–3.

Waller DA. Obstacles to the treatment of Munchausen by proxy syndrome. *Journal American Academy of Child and Adolescent Psychiatry.* 1983; **22**(1): 80–5.

Waring WW. The persistent parent. *American Journal of Diseases in Childhood.* 1992; **146:** 753–6.

Warner JO, Hathaway MJ. The allergic form of Meadow's syndrome (Munchausen by proxy). *Archives of Disease in Childhood.* 1984; **59**(2): 151–6.

Watson JBG, Davies JM, Hunter JLP. Non-accidental poisoning in childhood. *Archives of Disease in Childhood.* 1979; **54**(2): 143–4.

Whelan-Williams S, Baker T. A multidisciplinary hospital response protocol. In: Parnell TF, Day DO, editors. *Munchausen Syndrome by Proxy: misunderstood child abuse.* Thousand Oaks: Sage; 1998.

White ST, Voter K, Perry J. Surreptitious warfarin ingestion. *Child Abuse and Neglect.* 1985; **9**(3): 349–52.

Wood PR, Fowlkes J, Holden P, Casto D. Fever of unknown origin for six years: Munchausen syndrome by proxy (clinical conference). *Journal of Family Practice.* 1989; **28:** 391–5.

Woollcott P, Aceto T, Rutt C, Bloom M, Glick R. Doctor shopping with the child as proxy patient: a variant of child abuse. *Journal of Pediatrics.* 1982; **101**(2): 297–301.

World Health Organization. *ICD-10 Classification of Mental and Behavioural Disorders.* Geneva: World Health Organization; 1992.

Zohar Y, Avidan G, Shvili Y, Laurian N. Otolaryngologic cases of Munchausen's syndrome. *Laryngoscope.* 1987; **97**(2): 201–3.

Appendix

ICD and DSM terms for Dissociative and Somatoform Disorders

In the following pages two parallel systems for classifying **soma-tizing disorders** are presented as summary lists of the two major systems for the classification of psychiatric disorders; these are the ICD-10 and the DSM-IV (*see* Glossary). Although it is the ICD that is in use in the UK and Europe, both systems are presented because a substantial quantity of the literature comes from the USA. These systems are designed to be a tool for psychiatrists and are presented here as a source of reference for the reader who wishes to quickly see where a term they encounter may be found. One could consider them to be an outline map only. For any depth of information it will be necessary to refer to the full publications which are referenced. On the following pages is a little more detail, in the form of criteria, for elaborated and Factitious Disorders in both systems.

The ICD-10 classification

F44   Dissociative (Conversion) Disorders
F44.0   Dissociative Amnesia
F44.1   Dissociative Fugue
F44.2   Dissociative Stupor
F44.3   Trance and Possession Disorders
F44.4   Dissociative Motor Disorders
F44.5   Dissociative Convulsions
F44.6   Dissociative Anaesthesia and Sensory Loss
F44.7   Mixed Dissociative (Conversion) Disorders
F44.8   Other Dissociative (Conversion) Disorders
        .80 Ganser's Syndrome
        .81 Multiple Personality Disorder
        .82 Transient Dissociative (Conversion) Disorders Occurring in Childhood and Adolescence
        .88 Other Specified Dissociative (Conversion) Disorders
F44.9   Dissociative (Conversion) Disorder, Unspecified

F45	**Somatoform Disorders**
F45.0	Somatization Disorder
F45.1	Undifferentiated Somatoform Disorder
F45.2	Hypochondriacal Disorder
F45.3	Somatoform Autonomic Dysfunction (+ 6 organ system subtypes)
F45.4	Persistent Somatoform Pain Disorder
F45.8	Other Somatoform Disorders
F45.9	Somatoform Disorder, unspecified

F68	**Other Disorders of adult personality and behaviour**
F68.0	Elaboration of physical symptoms for psychological reasons
F68.1	Intentional production or feigning of symptoms or disabilities, either physical or psychological [Factitious Disorder]

The DSM-IV classification

Factitious Disorders

300.xx	Factitious Disorder (subtypes listed on pages 129–30)
300.19	Factitious Disorder NOS (includes the by proxy variant)

Somatoform Disorders

300.81	Somatization Disorder
300.81	Undifferentiated Somatoform Disorder
300.11	Conversion Disorder
307.xx	Pain Disorder (with subtypes)
300.7	Hypochondriasis
300.7	Body Dysmorphic Disorder
300.81	Somatoform Disorder NOS

Dissociative Disorders

300.12	Dissociative Amnesia
300.13	Dissociative Fugue
300.14	Dissociative Identity Disorder
300.6	Depersonalization Disorder
300.15	Dissociative Disorder NOS

Criteria for elaborated and Factitious Disorders

ICD-10 diagnostic criteria for research

F68.0 Elaboration of physical symptoms for psychological reasons

A Physical symptoms originally due to a confirmed physical disorder, disease, or disability become exaggerated or prolonged in excess of what can be explained by the physical disorder itself.

B There is evidence for a psychological causation for the excess symptoms (such as evident fear of disability or death, possible financial compensation, disappointment at the standard of care experienced).

F68.1 Intentional production of feigning of symptoms or disabilities, either physical or psychological [Factitious Disorder]

A The individual exhibits a persistent pattern of intentional production or feigning of symptoms and/or self-infliction of wounds in order to produce symptoms.

B No evidence can be found for an external motivation such as financial compensation, escape from danger, or more medical care. (If such evidence is found, category Z76.5, malingering, should be used.)

C (Most commonly used exclusion clause.) There is no confirmed physical or mental disorder that could explain the symptoms.

DSM-IV diagnostic criteria for Factitious Disorder

A   Intentional production or feigning of physical or psychological signs or symptoms.

B   The motivation for the behaviour is to assume the sick role.

C   External incentives for the behaviour (such as economic gain, avoiding legal responsibility, or improving well-being, as in malingering) are absent.

The code is then based on the type:

300.16   **With predominantly psychological signs and symptoms:**
if psychological signs and symptoms predominate in the clinical presentation.

300.19   **With predominantly physical signs and symptoms:**
if physical signs and symptoms predominate in the clinical presentation.

300.19   **With combined psychological and physical signs and symptoms:**
if both psychological and physical signs and symptoms are present but neither predominates in the clinical presentation.

Glossary

Assessment framework
The *Framework for the Assessment of Children in Need and Their Families* (Department of Health *et al.*, 2000) was introduced to promote a systematic approach to the assessment process and record keeping. The Framework in the Government Guidance was developed from legislative foundations together with an extensive research and practice knowledge. The now familiar triangle or pyramid is used to represent the three inter-related domains or systems: child's developmental needs, parenting capacity, and family and environmental factors. Each of these is contributed to by a number of critical dimensions. The impact of the Framework was reported in *Assessing Children's Needs and Circumstances: the impact of the Assessment Framework* (Department of Health, 2003).

Attachment theories
Developed by John Bowlby from 1958; fundamental aspects of human behaviour; deals with affectional bonds in terms of certain pre-programmed patterns of behaviour becoming focused upon another individual, which brings the individuals into emotional proximity and maintains this situation. The range of behaviours and emotions that may be considered when bonds are being made, broken, or threatened is wide. The theory looks at the phenomenon of attachment of one person with another meeting a biological need. When the attachment needs of an individual are not met, one effect may be to increase varieties of abnormal illness behaviour as a way of attempting to meet this powerful need. In extreme cases fabrication of illness may occur. In FII it is hypothesized that the fabricating mother has unmet attachment needs which primarily affect the attachment to her child and secondarily there is a pathological attempted attachment to doctors or medical services. A serious problem in the mother–child relationship may be well concealed by the focus on matters of illness.

CAMHS: Child and Adolescent Mental Health Service

A multi-disciplinary team, part of the NHS, offering assessment and therapies for children, adolescents and their parents – present in each health area of the UK. The team usually consists of psychiatrists, psychologists, nurses, family therapists, psychotherapists, and occupational therapists. The interventions offered include individual, family and group therapies, as well as medication for specific conditions.

Covert Video Surveillance (CVS)

'CVS should be used if there is no alternative way of obtaining information which will explain the child's signs and symptoms, and the multi-agency strategy discussion meeting considers that its use is justified based on the medical information available.' *See* Chapter 6 in *Safeguarding Children in Whom Illness is Fabricated or Induced* (HM Government, 2007), in particular the section on 'Use of Covert Video Surveillance'.

Critical path

A concept introduced by Lynch, which recognizes that a series of inter-related events leads to the final catastrophic event of the physical abuse of a child. Risk factors were identified and all contribute to the final situation in a holistic way. This is a forerunner of the 'ecological model'.

'Designated doctor' and 'designated nurse'

The terms **designated** and **named** professionals denote professionals with specific roles and responsibilities for safeguarding children. All PCTs should have a designated doctor and nurse to take a strategic, professional lead on all aspects of the health service contribution to safeguarding children across the PCT area, which includes all providers. Designated professionals are a vital source of professional advice on safeguarding children's matters to other professionals, the PCT, Local Authority children's services departments and the LSCB (HM Government, *Working Together to Safeguard Children*, 2006).

See also 'named doctor' and 'named nurse'.

Diagnostic and Statistical Manual of the American Psychiatric Association (DSM-IV): fourth edition
A comprehensive manual published by the American Psychiatric Association for use by mental health professionals. The purpose is to provide practical and useful advice for clinicians and it lists all psychiatric disorders with diagnostic criteria and other features of disorders such as prevalence, course and associated features.

Ecological model
A framework used by many clinicians and researchers for considering a wide range of aetiological factors which contribute to a situation in which child abuse occurs. The origins are from the work of Belsky (1980). The ecological model considers the child within the context of the family and the wider context of society and thus fits with the Assessment Framework (*see* above).

Factitious Disorder
A term used to refer to physical or psychological symptoms that are fabricated by an individual, either by verbally fabricating an account of various symptoms or with the addition of actually producing physical signs (thus causing some degree of self harm). The intention of the fabricator is to assume the sick role, rather than to achieve a clear goal such as financial gain or, classically, to avoid military conscription.

The term refers to a disorder in the DSM-IV with the subtypes of 'predominantly psychological signs and symptoms' and 'predominantly physical signs and symptoms', and a 'combined type'. The disorder may be limited to one or more brief episodes although it is often a chronic or at least a recurring problem.

The term is also a disorder in the ICD-10 listed as 'Intentional production or feigning of symptoms or disabilities, either physical or psychological'. A milder disorder is 'Elaboration of physical symptoms for psychological reasons'.

Factitious Disorder by Proxy
A term in the DSM-IV 'for further study' referring to the adult fabricator in the FII situation, i.e. similar to the Factitious Disorder but the fabrication is in another person. The term is not presently recommended.

Faltering growth
Formerly referred to as **failure to thrive (FTT)**.

Recent research has clarified the nature of faltering growth and a considerable knowledge base is available regarding contributory factors and interventions. Faltering growth is the term applicable when a child's weight falls significantly below the appropriate growth curve. The most cited factor contributing to faltering growth is difficulties in feeding and most cases do not have an organic cause. The faltering growth occurs because the child does not receive sufficient calories. Faltering growth occurs across all socio-economic groups.

Only a tiny minority of children fail to grow because of abuse or neglect; however, rare situations have been reported in which the child is deliberately fed too little in association with fabrication of illness; it may therefore occur as a rare form of **illness induction**.

(For more information about faltering growth *see* the *Professional Briefing Paper* by Angela Underdown and Eileen Birks (published by The Children's Society).)

Histrionic Personality Disorder
A disorder listed in the **ICD-10** characterized by:

* self-dramatization, theatricality, exaggerated expression of emotions
* suggestibility, easily influenced by others or by circumstances
* shallow and labile affectivity
* continual seeking for excitement, appreciation by others and activities in which the patient is the centre of attention
* inappropriate seductiveness in appearance and behaviour
* over-concerns with physical attractiveness.

Hysteria – Dissociative (conversion) disorder
The use of the term hysteria or conversion hysteria is now not recommended. According to the ICD-10 the Dissociative Disorders result from a partial or complete loss of the normal integration between memories of the past, awareness of identity and immediate sensations, and control of bodily movements. The dissociative motor disorders are perhaps the most evident with a partial or complete inability to use a limb, an inability to speak or

complete paralysis. The psychological mechanism is unconscious, by contrast with malingering, which is conscious and purposeful.

ICD-10: International Classification of Disease

Published by the World Health Organization and includes a classification of mental and behavioural disorders. It is the official classification system in the UK used by psychiatrists.

Illness behaviour

Illness behaviour refers to how people think and behave when they are, or think they are, or might be ill. Mechanic (1962), a sociologist, approached the subject of illness behaviour from the perspective of public health and medical sociology. The concept of *illness behaviour* was proposed, by which Mechanic referred to 'the ways in which given symptoms may be differentially perceived, evaluated and acted upon (or not acted upon) by different types of persons'. Although the term *illness behaviour* is not a clinical diagnosis, it may be considered useful by clinicians. By contrast ...

    Abnormal illness behaviour (abnormal behaviour in seeking healthcare) was defined by Pilowsky (1989) as 'the persistence of an inappropriate or maladaptive mode of perceiving, evaluating or acting in relation to one's own state of health, despite the fact that a doctor (or other appropriate social agent) has offered an accurate and reasonably lucid explanation of the nature of the illness and appropriate course of management to be followed (if any) with opportunities for discussion, negotiation and clarification based on adequate assessment of all biological, psychological, social and cultural factors'. Pilowsky started from the position of the physician who faces a patient with physical complaints for which no adequate organic cause can be found. A range of possible (psychiatric) diagnostic labels may be applied in such a situation. The importance of the explanation offered by the doctor raises the questions of accuracy and lucidity in the context of a matching between the understanding of the doctor and of the patient. For example, problems may arise if there are significant differences in the use of language, intellect, ethnicity and culture, especially if these differences are poorly appreciated by the doctor.

Inappropriate use of medication

Appropriate, or inappropriate, use of medication in young children is determined by the parent, who acquires and administers the medication. Inappropriate use may include excessive administration of medicines with a sedative action. If not prescribed for the child by a doctor, the medicines may be prescribed for another person, or obtained over the counter from the pharmacy. In the unusual situation of the administration being excessive the situation of toxicity or poisoning may result and may be associated with a fabrication of illness with induction of physical signs due to the medicine administered. A history of inappropriate medication was noted to have occurred in some of the families in which fabrication of illness had been identified by Bools *et al*. Administered medicine to excess may be difficult to differentiate from a child accidentally ingesting a medicine.

Induction of illness (production of signs)

The most immediately dangerous type of fabricated illness has occurred when children have been suffocated to induce a state similar to a seizure. Poisoning, usually with prescribed medicines, and withholding of nutrients have also been reported. The dilution of baby milk has been reported as a method of covertly withholding nutrition.

Infanticide

In 1938 a revision of the 1922 Infanticide Act defined *infanticide* as the killing of a child under 12 months. The mental state of the mother was defined in these terms. 'At the time of the act or omission the balance of her mind was disturbed by reason of her not having fully recovered from the effects of giving birth to the child or by reason of the effect of lactation consequent upon the birth of the child.'

Local Safeguarding Children Board: LSCB

In April 2006 the ACPC was replaced by the LSCB as required by the Children Act 2004. The LSCB is the key statutory mechanism for agreeing how the relevant organizations in each local area will cooperate to safeguard and promote the welfare of children in that locality, and for ensuring the effectiveness of what they do. The work of the LSCBs is part of the wider context of children's trust arrangements that aim to improve the overall well-being of all children in the local area (i.e. the five *Every Child Matters* outcomes). Whilst the work of the LSCB contributes to the wider goals of improving the well-being of all children, it has a particular focus on aspects of the 'staying safe' outcome. Details of the role, objectives and functions of the LSCB are set out in Chapter 3 of *Working Together to Safeguard Children* (HM Government, 2006).

Medical neglect

According to Erickson and Egeland in Chapter 1 of *The APSAC Handbook on Child Maltreatment* (American Professional Society on the Abuse of Children, 1996) the term medical neglect refers to 'caregivers' failure to provide prescribed medical treatment for their children, including required immunizations, prescribed medication, recommended surgery, or other intervention in the case of serious disease or injury'. The issue of whether neglect is, or is not, occurring may be complicated by differences of opinion between caregivers and the child's doctor, perhaps as a result of religious beliefs. However, the problem is addressed here because medical neglect may accompany FII and be one part of serious difficulties in providing adequate parenting. See Figure 5.3, page 67, *The spectrum of parental healthcare seeking by parents for their children* described by Eminson and Postlethwaite (1992), one element of which is *medical neglect*.

Munchausen Syndrome

Named by physician Richard Asher in 1951 to refer to a group of adults who presented themselves as patients to doctors, by falsifying symptoms and signs of illness. The behaviour was repeated, sometimes to the extent of almost becoming a lifestyle. The assumed objective of the behaviour was to assume the *sick role* including the desire to be admitted to hospital. Asher chose the name because he observed that like the famous *Baron Von Munchausen* the persons affected travelled widely and their stories were dramatic and untruthful. The modern, preferred, terminology is *Chronic Factitious Disorder*, which is a diagnosis found in the DSM and the ICD.

Munchausen Syndrome by Proxy

Following in the tradition of naming medical syndromes (a syndrome is a concurrence of several symptoms in a disease), the term *Munchausen Syndrome by Proxy* (or *MSP*) was first used in the UK by Meadow in 1976, derived from the term *Munchausen Syndrome*. Sometimes the term has been misused and perhaps the most misleading misuse of the term was to refer to a perpetrator of FII as 'suffering from *MSP*'. This confused many people and together with the overuse of the term *Munchausen Syndrome* and the relative complexity of the *by proxy* situation (with three elements of: the fabricating behaviour, the impact on the child of what is likely to be considered to be abuse, and the psychiatric status of the perpetrator) it was recommended that the term be abandoned, and the term FII be used. However, since the term *MSP* has been used since 1976 and still is used, notably at present in the United States, it remains necessary to keep the term in mind when reading literature and particularly including carrying out a search of the literature.

'Named doctor' and 'named nurse'

All NHS Trusts, NHS Foundation Trusts, and PCTs providing services for children should identify a named doctor and a named nurse/midwife for safeguarding. The named doctor and nurse should have expertise in children's health and development, child maltreatment, and local arrangements for safeguarding children and promoting their welfare (HM Government, *Working Together to Safeguard Children*, 2006).

Outlandish Factitious Disorder

A term used by Taylor to refer to the situation in which parents lay claim to a particular illness 'which is fashionable although controversial and for which there is no available refutable test'. The illness is not caused by the parents; however, the parents deeply hold beliefs about illness and the behaviour and beliefs of the child become subordinate to their parents' beliefs.

Pediatric Condition Fabrication (PCF)

A term suggested by APSAC (Munchausen Syndrome by Proxy task force of the American Professional Society on the Abuse of Children), which they define as 'a form of child maltreatment in which an adult falsifies physical and/or psychological signs and/or symptoms in a victim causing the victim to be regarded as ill or impaired by others. It is a sub-group of the *abuse by condition falsification* category of victimization in which the victim is another individual, adult or child'.

Poisoning

A method of *illness induction*: the production of physical signs in the child in conjunction with *verbal fabrication*. The *Oxford English Dictionary* states that a poison is 'any substance which, when introduced into or absorbed by a living organism, destroys life or injures health; popularly applied to a substance which destroys life by rapid action and when taken in a small quantity' (*Shorter Oxford English Dictionary*, 1980).

Pseudologia fantastica

This is a term used by psychiatrists to refer to what Simms (1988) calls the condition of 'fluent plausible lying' in which the un-truthful statements are often grandiose and extreme. The teller appears to believe in the fantastic statements. The condition is probably rather unusual and typically will occur when a person with a disordered personality, of a histrionic or asocial type, encounters a serious life crisis. The presentation is likely to be in the emergency department of a large hospital out of hours.

Sick role

A term introduced by the sociologist Talcott Parsons referring to the role which a person takes when they are suffering, or claim to be suffering, from an illness. The role is recognized by society and places certain obligations and privileges upon the incumbent. The privileges include exemption from normal duties and being taken care of by others. The obligations include having a desire to get well and to seek technically competent help in order to attempt to achieve this. This sociological perspective recognises the influence of aspects of the society on both the person in the sick role and the doctor within his/her culture of medical practice.

Significant harm

The Children Act 1989 introduced the concept of *significant harm*, and this is fully discussed with implications in *Significant Harm: its management and outcome* (2nd edition, Adcock and White, 1998). Significant is not defined in the Act; however, in the above publication, Richard White draws attention to the *Oxford English Dictionary* definition which is 'considerable, noteworthy or important'. *Harm* is defined in section 31(9) as *ill treatment* or the impairment of *health* or *development*. *Ill treatment* is defined as including sexual abuse and *forms of ill treatment which are not physical*, though it must by implication include physical abuse. *Health* is defined as physical or mental health. *Development* is defined as physical, intellectual, emotional, social or behavioural development. Children who have or are likely to have impaired health or development come within the definition of children in need.

(*See* 'The concept of significant harm', paragraphs 1.23–1.28 in *Working Together to Safeguard Children*, HM Government, 2006.)

Somatization
Somatization has been defined as 'the expression of personal and social distress in an idiom of bodily complaints with medical help seeking' (Kleinman and Kleinman, 1985).

Somatization Disorder
This is one of the *Somatoform Disorders* described in the ICD-10. The main features of *Somatization Disorder* are 'multiple, recurrent, and frequently changing physical symptoms, which have usually been present for several years before the patient is referred to a psychiatrist. Most patients have a long and complicated history of contact with both primary and specialist medical services, during which many negative investigations or fruitless operations may have been carried out'.

Somatizing
A descriptive term referring to the process of *somatization* (*see* definition above) in an individual.

Somatoform Disorders
In the ICD-10 (*see* above) the main feature of the *Somatoform Disorders* 'is the repeated presentation of physical symptoms, together with persistent requests for medical investigations, in spite of repeated negative findings and reassurances by doctors

that the symptoms have no physical basis. If any physical disorders are present, they do not explain the nature and extent of the symptoms or the distress and preoccupation of the patient'. A number of more specific diagnoses are listed under this category: Somatization Disorder, Undifferentiated Somatoform Disorder, Hypochondriacal Disorder, Somatoform Autonomic Dysfunction and Persistent Somatoform Pain Disorder.

Strategy discussion
Whenever there is reasonable cause to suspect that a child may be suffering, or is likely to suffer, significant harm, there should be a *strategy discussion*. The participants will be the Local Authority children's social care (who will be the conveners) and the police with other bodies as appropriate. If the child is a hospital patient the consultant should be involved and if an inpatient the senior nurse from the ward. The purposes and relevant matters are detailed in *Working Together to Safeguard Children* (HM Government, 2006), sections 5.54–5.59.

Symptom coaching
Defined by Sanders (1995) as 'the invitation the parent may give to the child to participate in symptom production'. Depending on the age of the child, and a number of other factors, the child may collude along a continuum with four points described as: naivety, passive acceptance, active participation and active harm. In the latter two points on the continuum the collusion is with the production of *physical signs* in addition to symptoms.

Verbal fabrication of symptoms
The essential feature of FII is the *verbal fabrication* of symptoms, which may be accompanied by enhancement of the story by falsification of specimens or records (charts), or by induction of physical signs.

Vulnerable child syndrome
This situation or 'syndrome' was first described by Green and Solnit in 1964, reviewed by Green in 1986 and more recently re-examined by Boyce in 1992. In this syndrome a mother becomes worried about potential illness in a child and subsequently overprotective because of fantasies she holds about the vulnerability

of the child, which may include that the child might die prematurely. The fantasies may have a variety of origins, such as an earlier serious illness, or psychological problems during, or after, the birth. The resulting difficulties forming the syndrome centre around pathological separation difficulties, infantilization, bodily over-concerns and for the child school under-achievement. In one form of the syndrome the mother has a psychological need to find something physically wrong with the child and repeatedly presents the child for medical attention.

Withholding nutrients/food
A method of *illness induction*, producing a poor state of health in a child, which may accompany a false story of various symptoms and a claim that physical illness is the cause of the symptoms. Withholding calories by the dilution of milk in the bottle for a baby is an example.

Index